EARTH and SPIRIT

Healing Lore and More from Puerto Rico

EARTH and SPIRIT

Healing Lore and More from Puerto Rico

María Dolores Hajosy Benedetti

Earth & Spirit: Healing Lore and More from Puerto Rico
also entitled
¡Hasta los baños te curan! Remedios caseros y mucho más de Puerto Rico

Published by
WATERFRONT PRESS
52 Maple Avenue
Maplewood, N.J. 07040

ISBN: 0-943862-46-9

Printed in the United States of America, 1989

para Puerto Rico, pasado, presente y futuro

Contents

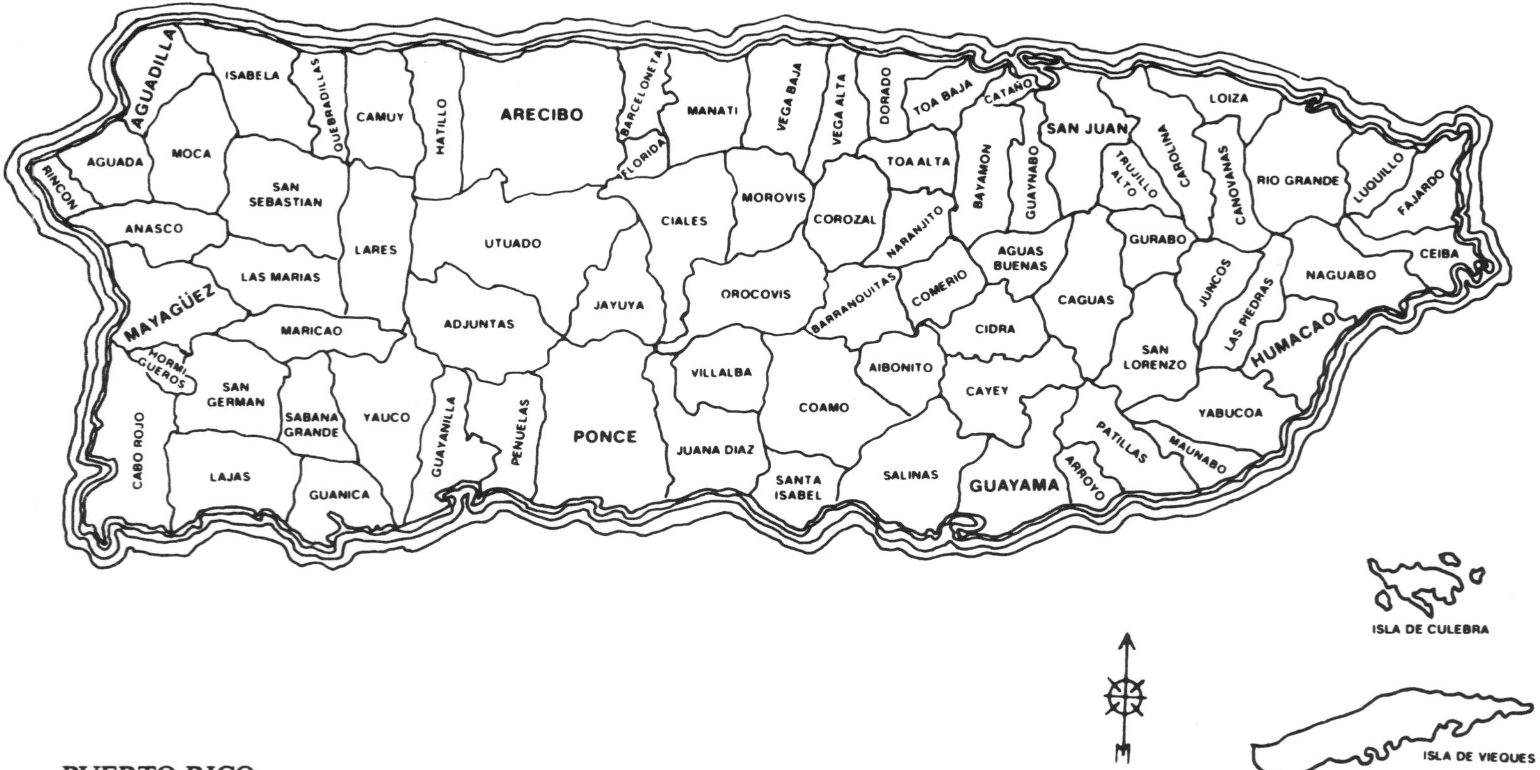

PUERTO RICO

Courtesy of Puerto Rico's Government Development Bank

The Power of the Past

a personal foreword

This book offers a glimpse of the tradition of popular medicine and related practices alive in Puerto Rico during the late 1980's: a system of mutual support and healing carried out by people close to their cultural roots.

This tradition of healing has arisen from real need, observation, experience, and respect—both for the individuals in need of healing, and for the environment which provides the tools and catalysts for that healing. And it survives because—on many levels and in many ways—it works.

* * *

The process of putting this book together has allowed me to explore and bring together two important aspects of my life: my love of nature and natural healing ways, and my Puerto Rican heritage which, too small a part of my childhood, I have begun to reclaim as an adult.

My grandmother's grandmother, Monserrate de Rivera, was a midwife in Mayagüez, Puerto Rico. Two generations later, my grandmother's sister, Librada Sotomayor Fernández, was an *espiritista** in the same town. She knew the medicinal plants,

* See glossary on p. 241 for definitions of italicized Spanish words.

counseled people according to her access to the spirit world, and healed children with stomach disorders through a type of spiritual massage called *santigüo*. It was Librada—my familial link here in New York with the old ways of Puerto Rico—who told me about the value of rue (*ruda*) for "female problems" and taught me to make a proper *sancocho*, "*como Dios manda.*" As I prepare now to move to her homeland, I thank her and my grandmother for reminding me of and connecting me with the power of the past.

* * *

When I was eight, I began working with diet and other natural methods of healing to treat serious allergies. Thanks to my father, my city-based childhood and adolescence were rich in rural experiences and early on, I fell in love with the natural world. When I was 17, I moved to the rural Catskill Mountain region of New York where, between college classes, I spent as much time as I could in the woods and fields exploring my spirituality and learning about plants. During eleven years of country living, I studied herbalism and shared information and experiences with friends involved with forms of medicine that not only cure disease but also nourish and strengthen. I worked with sound and color, a diet of whole foods, and wild plants that grew in my surroundings.

Why wild plants? For one thing, most pesticides used routinely on cultivated plants kill off not only insects (and people, if we're not careful) but also beneficial bacteria in the soil. These bacteria normally break down the elements of the earth and make them available to plants. Without these bacteria (and the chain of life that supports them) plants can not receive minerals from the soil and are made almost solely dependent upon the nitrogen, phosphorus and potash which are added to the earth in the form of commercial fertilizers. Nitrogen, phosphorus and potash may help plants to grow big and fast, but in terms of nourishment, the plants can't compete with their wild and organically grown counterparts, which ingest a wide range of minerals from non-contaminated soil.

Since we've evolved as a species eating and healing with wild plants for thousands and thousands of years, using wild plants also affirms our connection with our ancestors, and thus with the traditions that sustain and define us as a people . . . and as natural beings.

Finally, communion with the world of wild plants—using wild plants as food and medicine—is an ideal path to health maintenance, strengthening and healing because plants are a direct connection to the life force within and surrounding us all. This life force imbues the plants—and us—with the power to transform and thus, to heal.

Of course, as I learned from my mother and grandmother, the most effective medicine is often based on more than plant-related knowledge.

When I was growing up in Queens, New York, *abuelita* came often to care for my brother and me while my mother worked. And for 15 years, every single Wednesday, *abuela* cooked for us: *arroz con pollo, pollo con papas*, mouthwatering *rellenos de papa*, unforgettable *pasteles*, and once or twice a year, *arroz con coco*—that heavy-sweet, coconut-rice pudding with raisins, ginger, cinammon and bright, whole cloves. The ritual of eating this Puerto Rican soul food kept us sitting at the table for hours, savoring, remembering, laughing, arguing, planning, singing. On Wednesdays half the block smelled like *abuela's* food, and our kitchen was converted into a rollicking spiritual center.

Abuela's most memorable gift to us may have been physical nourishment, but she was also there for my brother and me when we were sick. She healed us as she rocked us on her lap, offered us teas of chamomile flowers, told us stories about Puerto Rico and tried desperately to teach us to iron. It was through *abuela* that I first became conscious of the relationship between love and the exercise of arduous quotidian chores (her way was always the long way, the slow way) and between healing and nourishment, always through love.

We are all healers. As long as we cook nourishing meals for one another, dance, sing and play music we love, use home remedies based on plants and other natural resources from our surroundings, ask for information from our dreams, pray or meditate, offer massages, and act intuitively on hundreds of other levels to keep ourselves healthy and correct imbalance, we are practicing medicine ways shared by traditional peoples all over the world.

Although certain people have always been recognized as having the "gift" of healing, traditional folk medicine is generally accessible to all. That is, regardless of economic and educational background, everyone can learn to use some useful, natural healing techniques. The work of most traditional healers is based upon nourishment on physical, emotional and spiritual levels, and upon an ability to transform through this nourishment. Few are specialists. Many work "full time" in other, unrelated fields. These factors contribute to traditional folk medicine's invisibility, but make it no less valuable.

Since the dawn of human society, traditional healers have worked in myriad ways to support the health and integrity of individuals, families and entire communities, while helping to maintain a balanced relationship between people and their environment. Even today, traditional folk healers tend to 80% of the world's entire population[1]. And all over the world, the

[1] From *The Hidden Power of Plants*, WGBH Educational Foundation, NOVA series, Public Television 1987.

practices of traditional midwives and healers—from shamans to bonesetters—are being validated through science.

Traditional peoples from Africa to Tibet to Greenland to the Americas have always recognized and made use of psychological and spiritual influences in medicine. During the last 25 years or so, post-industrial science has assured us that, yes, our own bodies can be stimulated by certain psychological states to produce the chemicals we need to feel and get better when we are depressed or ill. And the investigations have really just begun. Meanwhile, plants ranging from garlic to the fungus ergot (used by traditional healers and midwives all over the world) are being recognized and taken more and more seriously as valuable crude drugs and/or sources of highly valued oils and alkaloids, which serve as the basis of pharmaceutical preparations. In fact, several pharmaceutical companies are taking part in special research programs with the aim of finding drugs to treat cancer, AIDS, and herpes[2]. These programs involve working closely with traditional medical practitioners who have been using plants for generations, and who have established empirical evidence of success. In general, connections with folklore guarantee a high probability of finding active sub-

[2] According to the Herb Research Foundation *Herbalgram* #11, winter 1987, In 1987 The National Cancer Institute awarded five-year contracts to the New York Botanical Garden, the Missouri Botanical Garden, and the University of Illinois, respectively: $627,000 for plants from South America; $654,000 for plants from Africa; and $1.4 million for plants from Southeast Asia. The New York Botanical Garden will collect about 1500 specimens from Latin American tropical forests, especially those used medicinally by indigenous populations. The plants will be tested in extract form for anti-tumor activity.

Anti-herpes and anti-AIDS substances are also being sought in the same way with great interest. Plus, a natural insecticide is currently being sought to fight against the mosquito *Aedis egyptiae*, responsible for the spread of dengue and malaria.

stances. Also, as evidenced in this volume, traditional healers are likely to find not just one, but several uses for each "complex, crude drug specimen" (plant), while the academically-trained pharmacologist tends to investigate isolated compounds in search of one specific activity to counteract one particular health condition or narrowly related problems.

Several contributors to *Earth and Spirit* use plants whose value has not been proven by the scientific establishment. But there are many reasons for this. For instance, when science tests plants for their value as drugs, "non-active" constituents such as chlorophyll, glucosides and nutritive factors are ignored. In most cases, only alkaloids—which have the most dramatically observable biological effects—are sought, measured, and tested[3]. And while this approach has yielded many life saving drugs, it ignores the factors of *nourishment (wild*

[3] The process of isolating individual "active" constituents is described by Dr. Oswaldo Guerrero of the Department of Pharmaceutical Science at the University of Puerto Rico in Río Piedras:

"First, the plant must be collected and dried; we're not interested in the water content of the plant, and dried plants take up far less space than fresh ones. There are special drying ovens which allow for the process to take place slowly. Then, once they're dried, we powder the plant material and make extracts of the plant using solvents such as ethanol. The ethanol extracts all of the [alcohol solvent] plant's components. Then we evaporate the alcohol and we're left with an extract of the plant. It includes the plant's constituents in a small volume, which makes it very easy to work with.

"Next, the extracts are given to the pharmacologist or to the microbiologist—the scientist who can help us to determine if the plant has the activity we're looking for: diuretic, anti-diabetic, etc. The pharmacologist might use animals or micro-organisms to do the testing.

"Then we divide the extract into two solvents which have a different polarity, and using a process called chromatography, we separate the fractions even more. Then, when we present the fractions to the pharmacologist once more, we find out exactly what part is active and we separate that fraction from the others."

plants are extremely high in vitamins and minerals in a form that is optimally received and utilized by the body), the *tonifying effect* of plants taken over a long period of time, the often surprising *effects of combining plant substances*, and the *psychological-spiritual aspect* of working with local plants and a trusted healer. Of course, this last aspect of healing, although both unmeasurable and unproveable by objective means, is recognized and valued to varying degrees in every culture.

Through generations of experience and empirical testing, the people of Puerto Rico have made some astute and extremely important observations in terms of plant classification. For instance, designation of medicinal plants as "hot or cold" in their activity corresponds to two scientific categories, denoting the presence and absence of alkaloids. According to the observations of one Puerto Rican pharmacognosist, most "hot" plants are bitter. Containing alkaloids, their use should be controlled according to the knowledge of experienced herbal medicine practitioners. Many produce side effects. "Cooling" plants are more nourishing and refreshing. Many are diuretic. They can be taken on a regular basis, and are not bitter. "For this reason," he explains, "you'll note that 'hot' herbs are recommended for acute conditions, including fevers, and that 'cool' herbs are taken all the time."

Personally, I can attest to the efficacy of many of the remedies described in this work: aloe (*sábila*) for bronchial complaints, burns and constipation, wild balsam apple (*cundeamor*) for skin problems, chicken bone broth for chronic fatigue, rue (*ruda*) and broadleaf coriander (*recao*) for menstrual irregularity, and herbal baths for physical and spiritual renewal are among them.

And modern computer studies validate the tremendous knowledge and foresight shown by traditional farmers throughout the world, proving that practices like "planting with the moon" not only offer us superior nourishment, but also contribute greatly to the health of our environment.

Rich in practical knowledge and wisdom, the island's earth-based medicine tradition represents a tremendous contribution to the healing sciences, and to Puerto Rican and Caribbean culture. I hope that this small body of work will spark interest in the passing on of more and more information by word of mouth, songs, writings, and the growing practice of what we still remember.

Acknowledgements

This book has been written in gratitude to the people of Puerto Rico who, along with their knowledge, shared food, shelter, warmth, music and laughter with me along the way:

Edwin Aguayo, Rosa Ligia Alvarez, Petra Angleró, Mikhail Antoun, Ph.D., María Cruz Avilés, Félix Nicholás Beato, Beba, Alma and Roberto Cabán, la familia Carrer, Ana Clausells de Costoso, Carmen Colón de Jorge, Carlos Alberto Costoso, Pepe Chávez, Delia, Eusebio Díaz Díaz, Cecilia Fernández, Angel González, Ricardo Oswaldo Guerrero, Ph.D., María Lagoa de González, Irenio López Mercado, Tomás Luzcampos, Freddy Martell, Eliot Monteverde, Carmen María Morales Serrano, Panky Negrón Maldonado, Dr. Esteban Núñez Meléndez, Alida and Edgardo Ortiz, Ramona Ortiz Santana, Casimira Osoris Fuentes, María Otero Collazo viuda de Santiago, Altagracia Pagán, Rafaela Parrilla, Josefina Pizarro, Luisa Flores Rivera, Providencia Rivera, Barbara and Cheo Rodríguez, Kique and Tato Rodríguez Valentín, Carmen Rodríguez Vargas, Margarita Roque, Carmen Rupert, María Salgado, Cruz María Santiago, Eugenio Santiago Marrero, Julia Santiago, Marinilda Santini, Aida Sotomayor de Ramos, Brígida Sotomayor Vargas, Mercedes Sotomayor viuda de Martell, Tai, Unmilo, Paula Valentín Mercado, Vanessa, Brunilda Vargas Muñiz, Camila Vargas viuda de Sotomayor, Inés Vargas Muñiz, Primi Socorro Vargas, Carmen Vega, Victor, Yari.

Also, I offer sincere thanks to the following people for volunteering their editorial and moral support, for believing in the value of this project, and for, in many ways, helping me to bring it to fruition:

María Benedetti Hajosy, who read every interview in English and in Spanish, helped with difficult transcriptions, and whose love, music and ongoing support over 34 years made this book possible,
José Manuel Torres Santiago, who shares his love for and pride in his culture through classes, writings and public talks, and whose knowledge inspired my commitment to this project,
Jaime Antonio Estades Roque, who said, "Go! I know a few people there who will be glad to talk with you . . . ." and who offered essential feedback as I put this book together,
Pedro Acevedo Rodríguez, for checking botanical references and carefully reading the text,
Elmer Sánchez, for verifying congruence between taped and written material,
Kenneth Gumbs, for sharing his encyclopedic knowledge about Afro-caribbean music and religions,
Herminio Vallejo, for acting as cultural and linguistic consultant,
Librada Sotomayor Fernández, for her stories, cooking lessons, and love,
Melchia Crowne, for ongoing and essential wisdom and support,
Judith Vélez, for help with two difficult transcriptions,
Susun S. Weed, for her classes and writings since 1977,
Kal Wagenheim, for his editorial suggestions.

And finally, thanks to the circle of wholeness, the roads that opened, my protectors and guides, the music, the dreams, and the trees, who give of themselves so that we can read books.

The Medicine of Yesterday, Today

doña Paula Valentín Mercado and
Tato Rodríguez Valentín
of Las Marías

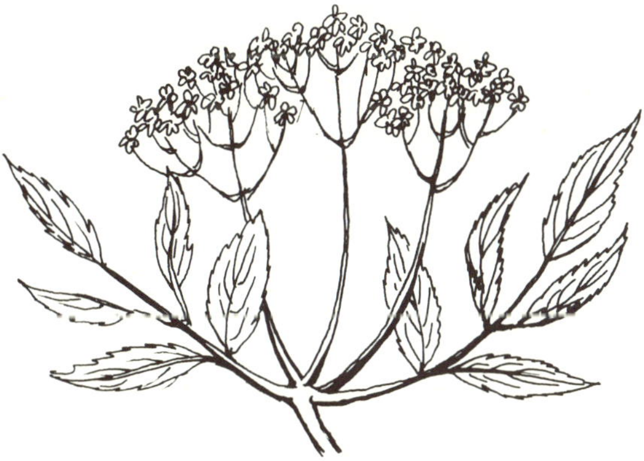

elder *el saúco*

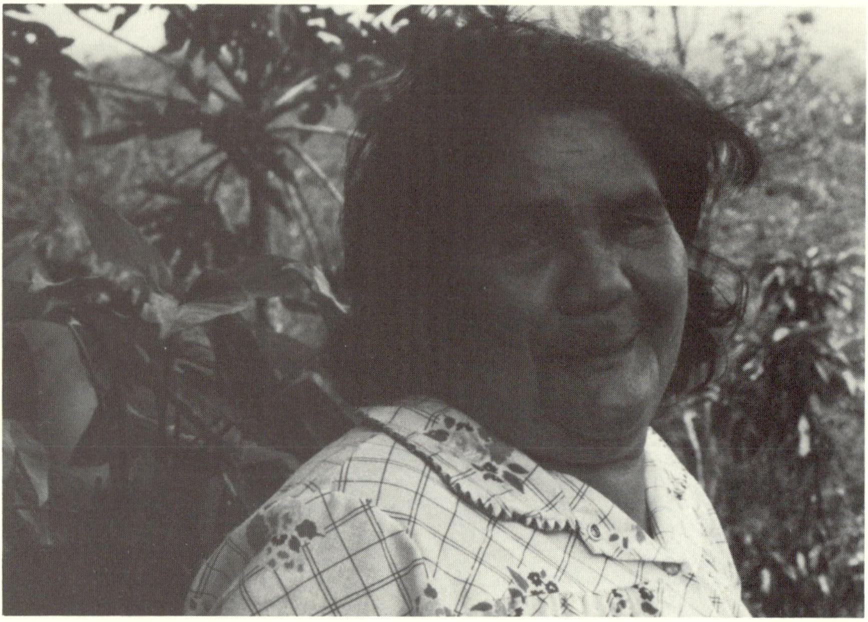

Paula Valentín Mercado

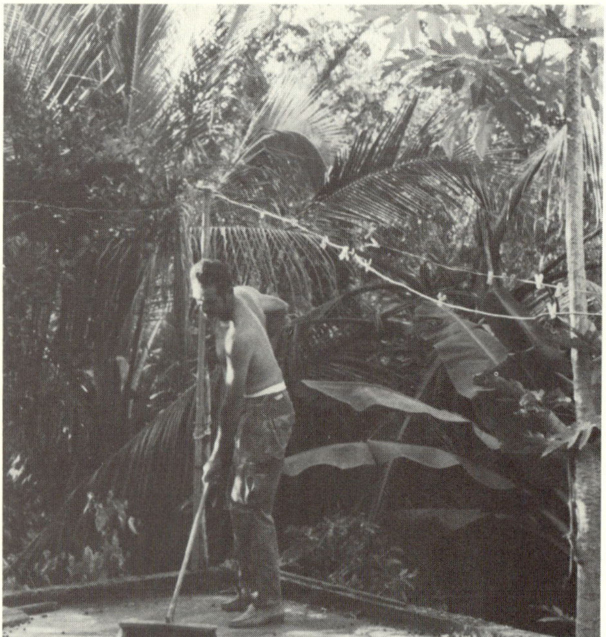

Tato Rodríguez Valentín, drying coffee

The Medicine of Yesterday, Today

doña Paula Valentín Mercado and Tato Rodríguez Valentín of Las Marías

My meeting with doña Paula took me by surprise. I had stopped the car outside of Las Marías to photograph her home, bordered by a native pine tree and several medicinal plants.

As I approached, I noticed the welcoming smell of a wood fire, and suddenly faced doña Paula as she trudged up the hill behind her house, wiping the sweat from her forehead with a well-worn handkerchief.

"What are you looking for?"

"I was hoping I could take a picture of your beautiful herbs. I'm interested in medicinal plants."

"Well, plants are my medicine. Pills make me feel horrible, so I use the plants, and I grow them right here."

"I'd love to hear about how you use herbs."

"At your service. But let's go inside and have something cold to drink first. Do you like pineapple juice?"

That's how it started.

I stayed for two days and two nights with doña Paula and her sons, eating rice with fresh native lentils (*gandules*) just picked off the bush, knocking papayas and oranges off the trees, climbing the nearby hills, separating small pebbles from the sun-dried coffee beans, watching a mountain sunrise and a

7 AM livestock sale, touring the road to Arecibo and all points in between, asking questions about plants and traditional agricultural practices, roaming the farm, drinking spring water from impromptu cups made from wide, green malanga leaves, and collecting leaves, stems, roots, and flower specimens for my book of pressed, medicinal plants. All this in the warm and familiar spirit of rural Puerto Rican hospitality.

Doña Paula raised six sons without moving even a mile away from her father's farm, where she grew up. In her life she's seen many dirt roads become paved ones, and many of her neighbors have moved to "the city." But where she lives in Las Marías, agriculture is still a source of livelihood for many, a source of pride for all.

Paula: I'm 71 years old, and I was born right below, at the lower edge of the farm here. My parents were simple *jíbaros*, and they dedicated themselves to cultivating the soil.

In those days, we all worked at embroidery and washed clothes for people; but most of all, we harvested coffee. And believe me, it wasn't easy. Back then, a 28-pound measure (*almúd*) of coffee was worth 15 cents! Anyway, that's how we grew up, always working. There were eleven of us kids.

They built a school nearby when I was ten years old, In order to get there, I had to cross the river and walk along roads which were really just mud paths. I made it through the third grade when I was 14. Then I started working full-time on the farm and at a neighbor's house.

M: What do you like most about living in the country?

Paula: I love the plants and the animals. I've always raised cows and chickens, for instance. We have 18 chickens, a bunch of chicks, and three baby roosters that have already begun to crow. We also have cows and calves, and they provide fertilizer for the plants. Country life gives me a great deal of satisfaction.

M: I was attracted to your home by the medicinal plants growing outside. Can you talk about some of them?

Paula: Well, I have *paletaria. Paletaria* tea is cooling and very good for children when they get heat rash and other skin irritations. *Paletaria* tea is also good for bladder problems, especially when someone has difficulty urinating. It's very cooling.

A strong tea of rue (*ruda*) is also good for painful urination and bladder problems but, like fennel (*hinojo*), it's most well known for women's monthly cramps and related conditions.

Here we have lemon balm (*toronjil*) and red mint (*yerba buena*). They're both very good for the stomach. If you're nauseous and vomiting, you just need a good tea of the two combined. I'll tell you, that lemon balm is the best thing in the world, but if there's none around, you can also use sour orange leaves (*hoja de naranjo*).

M: You use these remedies frequently?

Paula: Whenever I need them. The plants are my medicine. Look, there's a highly medicinal plant, black nightshade (*mata gallina*). It makes a good tea mixed with Caribbean vervain (*la verbena*) for fever. Black nightshade and *paletaria* grow all over the place! And look over there; that spineless (*tuna*) cactus is great chopped up and boiled for a while. It's nourishing and it's also good for stomach problems.

I had some beautiful *yerba Luisa* and marjoram (*mejorana*) too, but once I had to travel, and when I returned, people had come by and they'd taken the plants that were just budding. You see, people today just don't know how to work with plants. For example, few people know that *yerba Luisa* should only be picked during the cool of the morning.

We walk toward the back yard, which offers a view of the mountainous, green countryside below and beyond us.

Paula: Here we have the coffee. I plant it, I harvest it, I dry it, I toast it on the wood stove, then I drink it. And I love it! I have cans of coffee there waiting to be toasted, but I only do that work in the cool of the morning. Otherwise I get a terrible headache.

Doña Paula points to an old fashioned, outdoor woodburning stove.

M: You don't see too many stoves like that one any more. The fire wood smells wonderful.

Paula: Yes, here I toast my coffee and cook up the root vegetables (*viandas*) and beans. I also prepare food for the pig here. I use my outdoor stove for the most difficult cooking chores. When you came along, I was cooking beans for dinner.

M: How did you learn everything you know about medicinal plants?

Paula: From my mother. When I was a child, we never bought medicines. We always used the plants from the earth. Whenever we got sick, *mamá* made remedies from whatever was growing. She used orange leaves (*naranjo*) and elder (*saúco*) a lot, for instance. And I still use them. You just boil up the beautiful white elder flower with some orange leaves and ginger (*jengibre dulce*), and that tea takes away your cold. We used to make that and many other medicines from boiled plants. We usually added honey, which is the best thing in the world.

For cold and congestion we also used strong teas or *guarapos* of *poleo*.

M: And for fevers?

Paula: For fever we used a *guarapo* of Caribbean vervain and common plantain (*llantén*). Lemon grass (*limoncillo*) also lowers fever. My mother used to peel and mash up the lemon grass root, and then boil it up with anise seeds (*anís*). We'd drink that tea hot when we had fever, and no matter how high the fever, it worked.

M: Lemon grass has such a beautiful fragrance.

Paula: And it's so useful. You can even brush your teeth with the root. You make a little package with it and just pass it over your gums as if it were a toothbrush. It freshens up the breath and makes your mouth feel great.

But before I get off the subject of fever, you can also take the leaves of bitter orange and add *poleo* and yellow elder (*saúco amarillo*). That *guarapo* cools the fever and gets rid of even the worst cough in the world.

For fever and headache, we always used *salvia*. For a simple headache, we might just tie warmed-up leaves on to our forehead and temples with a handkerchief. For fever, we would stick *salvia* leaves to the soles of our feet with camphor (*alcanfor*) cream and stick more leaves on to our foreheads.

In the U.S. you probably don't see too many of these home remedies, but here we grew up harvesting coffee and planting native fruits. We were always enduring the heat of the sun, and we got tremendous headaches. That's why we used the *salvia* leaves so often.

I get headaches nowadays too, but it's from high blood pressure.

M: How do you treat high blood pressure?

Paula: When passion fruit (*parcha*) is in season, I drink the juice. I've also heard that papaya lowers the blood pressure, but I've never tried it. I'll tell you one thing though, papaya mixed with grated coconut and boiled up with sugar makes one phenomenal dessert!

M: Are there some activities that seem to affect your blood pressure?

Paula: Well my headaches seem to be related to what I eat, and red meat seems to make them worse. When I have chamomile (*manzanilla*) I use it, and it helps me . . . and not only for headaches! It's also good for the stomach and for body aches and fever. Yes, chamomile helps me a lot. Here in Las Marías it flowers in December; by January it's already dry. I save the flowers that come in December for making my teas, because it's the best thing in the world. And you know, they sell it in drug stores and even the fancy stores too, nowadays.

If my headache is really bad, I'll put my feet in a big bucket of hot water. That treatment also lowers the blood pressure when I feel it's gone all the way up.

When I suffer from nerves, I make a tea of sour orange leaves and that helps a lot.

M: Have you ever sold any of the herbs you grow here?

Paula: No, but when people come looking for medicinal plants, I give them the remedies they ask for. In fact, just the other day a doctor from town came looking for some aloe vera (*sábila*). A child had been badly burned, and aloe is the best thing in the world for burns. First the doctor came, then the next day he sent his wife over here, and finally, they sent a little boy to get some more.

M: Do you know of any other uses for the aloe plant?

Paula: It's very good if someone has chest pains, and there are many ways of preparing it. My father used it a lot. First we peeled it, cut it up, and put it in a jug of water. Then we left it outside during the night, every night. During the day, he'd drink it. My father also suffered from sore throat and coughs, and he swore by aloe vera for those conditions too.

I'm always in the sun and I use aloe when my skin gets dried out and burned. I simply cut it and pass the inside gel over my skin as if it were a lotion. It's tremendous for the skin, really.

You know, when my father's kidney pains started in, we used to cut the fat leaves of the spineless tuna cactus into two flat slices. Then we cooked them among the coals for a while, and when they'd cooled off, we placed them on his lower back and covered it all with a towel. That helped him a lot.

I show her my book of the pressed plants I'm collecting.

Paula: Here you have *ipecacuana*. It's very good for coughs, and it can be used for children and grownups alike. You simply boil the green part with red mint or lemon balm or marjoram. It really gets rid of phlegm.

The castor bean plant (*higuereta*) is used to make poultices. We used to heat up the leaf, chop it up, mix it with belladonna ointment and then wrap it on swollen ankles. It was good for any kind of inflammation, including for the cows, when they were all swollen after giving birth.

They don't sell belladonna ointment anymore, but my mother also used it when someone had a toothache or other swellings of the mouth, even mumps.

And when someone suffered from arthritic joints, we rubbed the grease of a guinea hen on the joints as if it were lotion. My girl, there are so many home remedies!

M: I've heard that *cundeamor* is used for getting rid of fungus.

Paula: If you have a problem with itching, you simply boil it up and take a bath in it. The castor bean plant can be used in the same way, actually.

We come inside to separate stray pebbles from the dried coffee, and Tato, her eldest, 40's-ish son arrives. I show him my book of plant specimens, and spontaneously, the conversation resumes.

Tato: The boiled root of *moriviví* cured my brother when he had an infected molar. He swished mouthfuls of it around and the pain subsided completely. It worked right away, and his tooth hasn't bothered him since then at all.

Then there's *guaco*, which grows just about everywhere. A bath of *guaco* is good for open sores, cuts and many other conditions. It kills germs. In fact, there used to be a saying, when someone was beyond all help, "Not even *guaco* can save you." People had a lot of faith in that plant.

Paula: You know, I prepare ginger with hot milk at night when we have what we consider cold weather, and we do have cold weather in the mountains here. You simply mash up the ginger and boil it in a little bit of water for ten to fifteen minutes. Then you mix that water with hot milk and add sugar to taste. Delicious!

Ginger is tremendously warming, whether you take it internally or as a poultice. When my father suffered from leg cramps, my mother prepared bitter ginger (*jengibre amargo*) this way: First she would heat it up in the live coals. When it got soft, she'd take it out and let it cool. Then she'd mash it up and put it in the *alcoholado* for rubs. She used two or three handfuls of ginger per litre of *alcoholado*, which got stronger with time. Those ginger rubs really worked for him.

Tato: Ginger is also great for stomach cramps, or when you're just feeling weak. It stimulates the circulation. And we've always used it for therapeutic baths.

M: Can you describe one of those baths?

Tato: First you find the leaves and roots you want to use: Caribbean vervain, castor bean leaves, *higuillo oloroso*, *rompecota*, ginger, a little bit of everything. We use about three small handfuls for five gallons of water, and you boil the plants for a good half hour so that their medicinal qualities can be transferred to the water.

Paula: Then, when that liquid is no longer too hot, you wash up and then you have someone pour that bath over your entire body. The running stream of water takes away body pains and other bad feelings.

Tato: After the bath, you can't rinse yourself off or anything, because you don't want to dilute the benefits of the plants. The best thing about these baths is that they wash away both physical and mental complaints.

If someone has a fever, the same type of bath will help a great deal to lower it.

M: Tato, do you have a favorite plant?

Tato: Absolutely. The elder (*saúco*). For me it's the most beautiful flower in the world, and I've done a lot of travelling, seen a lot of flowers. I also admire it for its subtle fragrance.

M: I've enjoyed elder flowers as a food, fried up in batter like fritters. The berries are also wonderful. And the root of the elder tree is known around the world as a universal remedy. It's probably one of the most important medicinal plants available today.

Tato: I've used it for colds and fever, and you can drink teas of the flowers and leaves even if you're not sick. It's a beautiful plant!

Paula: Well, that's how it was, the medicine of yesterday. It worked for us then, and for some of us, it still does.

Doña Petra's Favorite Remedies

Petra Angleró
of Retirement Village

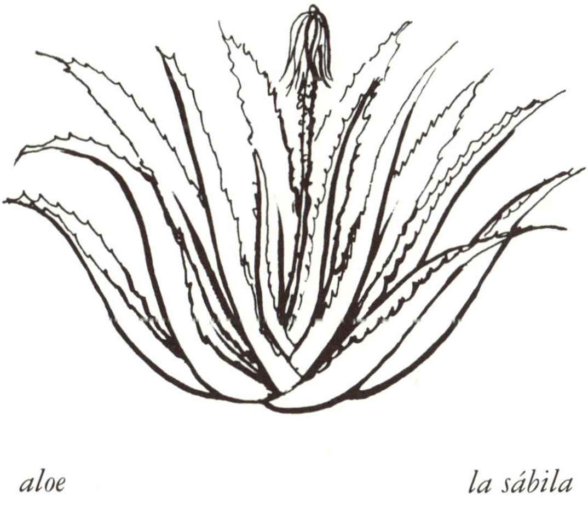

aloe *la sábila*

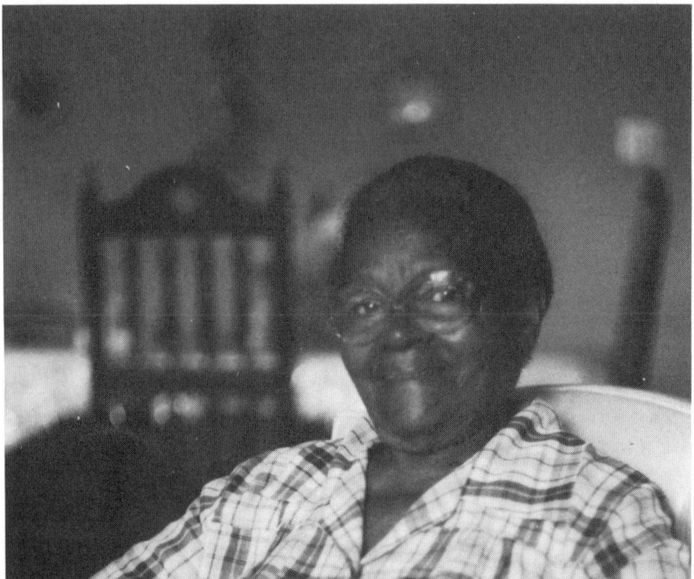

Petra Angleró

Doña Petra's Favorite Remedies

Petra Angleró
of Retirement Village

I met doña Petra Angleró in the Plaza Colón of Mayagüez during a nocturnal Holy Week procession. My cousin had told me, "Petra knows about plants that heal," and she was right. Doña Petra lives in a modern retirement condominium, where she is active in several community activities. She also serves as a member of the Legion of Mary, caring for the aged. Although she lives in the city, she stays close to the natural world through her house plants (aloe vera, violets, the "lucky" snake plant) and even through the presence of neighborly *reinitas,* small birds who drop in through her sunny balcony to snack on the sugar she leaves for them in her living room. She says her eyes are "bad" but from her sixth floor apartment, she pointed out little plants in the lot below that I couldn't distinguish even with my 20/20 vision. "It must be my affinity for them," she explained smiling.

Petra: I was born in Maricao, and that's where my mother, Felícita Ortiz, taught me all about plants. In those days, when we had asthma attacks, she would mash up the stems of elder (*saúco*) to extract the juice. For every two tablespoons of that juice, she would mix a teaspoon of cooking oil and a pinch of salt. We took it as often as she told us to, and within two or three days, no more asthma!

In those days, everyone recognized the value of the plants, but just look out that window. They just chopped down the biggest *malagueta* tree around. Nowadays people just don't take plants seriously. I don't know what they must be thinking. What could be more important than nature and the medicine that comes from nature?

M: I've been thinking a lot about the times when people didn't have access to hospitals as they do now. How did the people of Maricao deal with a broken arm or leg?

Petra: When I was growing up, we used to use a plant called Madeira vine (*sueldaconsuelda*). We heated the leaves up on the stove, chopped them up and mixed them in a little bowl with warm cooking oil. After the bone had been set, we put that Madeira vine poultice all over the affected area and covered it with gauze or other fabric. We would leave it for about two days before changing it, and it helped a lot. It was also very effective when used for sprains.

M: Have you used many plant-based poultices?

Petra: Sure. I've made many the way I just described, and I've made them by simply placing a leaf covered with ointment on top of the affected area and holding it on with a wrap of some kind. You can also mash a leaf until it gives its liquid, and put that liquid on top of the bruise or whatever it is. It depends on the problem you want to treat.

I prepare my own medicated camphor ointment to use with plant poultices. I take a five-ounce jar of Vaseline and I melt it in a little saucepan on a low flame. Then I mash two little blocks of camphor until they're just powder, and I add that powder to the Vaseline on the stove. When it's all dissolved, I let it cool a little and then I spoon it all back into the same Vaseline jar.

M: I'm especially interested in remedies which are made from foods. Do you know any?

Petra: The best remedy for a woman who has just given birth is what we call the calabash (*higüera*) or white gourd medicine. During birth, the uterus goes through a lot, and may even get displaced. The white gourd medicine nourishes and tonifies the womb at a time when it needs support. So with this remedy and a good rest, the mother will always be fine.

M: Do you cook up the gourd?

Petra: No, it's a type of tisane, so it's not cooked at all.

The traditional way of making it is this: First, bore a hole in one end of a large, unripe, white calabash and pour into that hole as many whole cloves (*clavo de especia*), anise seeds (*anís en grano*) and anise stars (*anís de estrella*) as fit into one's hand. Then, bury the gourd for a couple of days until a liquid forms inside. The spices keep it from going bad, but it does ferment a little.

If you want to be more modern, you can make the same medicine by scooping all of the flesh and seeds from the gourd, putting it in a glass bowl, adding the spices and leaving it in the refrigerator for a few days before offering it to the woman.

Any way it's prepared, she should take about a cup a day—liquid and solid—for about nine days straight. And during that time she should really rest. In fact, if she wants to preserve her womb, she shouldn't do any heavy work at all for a full 40 days! Today, so many modern women go back to work just a couple of weeks after giving birth.

M: A lot has changed.

Petra: Yes, but women still boil up the paper-like peel and ends of a couple of heads of garlic (*ajo*) to treat menstrual pains. And even now, if you have a fungus growth on your skin, the best remedy is a bottle of *cundeamor*. Simply fill a bottle with the chopped-up fresh plant, and cover it all with three parts cooking oil and one part rubbing alcohol. Then leave it for a few days so that the medicinal qualities and color of the plant can seep into the liquid, and apply it to the affected area as often as needed. You can get completely cured with that, and I guarantee it, because I have tried it.

M: And it's so easy to prepare!

Petra: It's only easy if there's *cundeamor* growing in your neighborhood!

M: I'm sitting here admiring your beautiful aloe vera (*sábila*) plant. Do you use it for medicine?

Petra: Come and see what I have in the refrigerator, so you can learn something new. With this aloe compound, I've relieved my grandson's asthma several times. Used to be he couldn't even sleep, coughing all the time. And his poor mother, running to the doctor at all hours of the night. That's when I started preparing him my aloe vera compound. But taste the raw aloe first.

M: It smells like underarm sweat, and it's *extremely* bitter!

Petra: OK, now taste my aloe compound. Most of the liquid you see here is from the aloe, which I'm letting steep with some honey and spices.

M: Mmmm. It tastes like cloves, spicy . . . almost hot, and it's lost its bitterness. Delicious! What's the recipe?

Petra: I begin with about a litre of aloe gel: that's the gel of about five or six large, fleshy leaves. I add a cup of honey and another cup of spices, like star anise, whole cloves and cinammon. Then I add a cup of rum to preserve it. Without the rum, some mold may grow on it . . . and I think the rum enhances the flavor too! (laughter) Then I wait ten days or two weeks before taking it, a tablespoon at a time. And listen, besides asthma, it's also good for indigestion.

M: Yesterday I interviewed three people, and after each interview, I was offered a full meal. I ate so much that this morning my stomach was a little edgy. I couldn't even eat breakfast. But this aloe compound seems to be helping already.

Petra: Look around for a little jar and take some with you, love. May it serve you, and may God bless you for me.

Midwife and Bonesetter of Orocovis

doña María Cruz Avilés

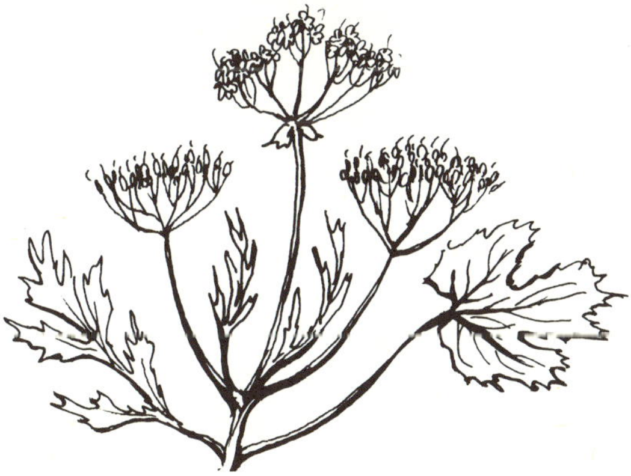

anise *el anís de semilla*

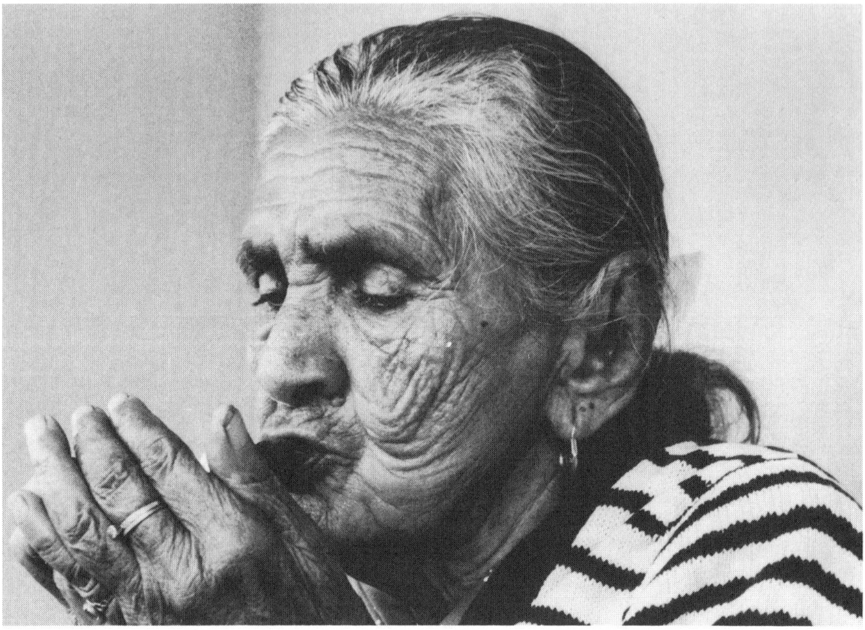

María Cruz Avilés

Midwife and Bonesetter of Orocovis

doña María Cruz Avilés

I arrived in Orocovis on Sunday, May 3, during the agricultural festival, so I had a chance to be surrounded by lots of people who love the land. I asked adults of all ages about traditional healers in the area, and almost everyone mentioned doña María Cruz.

"She helps the women give birth,"

"She sets bones,"

"She gives healing massage,"

"She's almost 90 years old now,"

"Everybody knows her,"

"She's my midwife,"

"If you pull a muscle, you can go to her,"

"If you break your arm . . . ."

"She helped deliver every child in my family."

The festival was small, but generous, and I gathered free samples of cacao, native pine saplings and regional fruits. There was excitement in the air, partly because later that night, Andrés Jiménez, Orocovis' own internationally famous troubador, would perform. With eight hours to wait before the concert, I was guided to the road to las Alturas, a low income project about two miles out of town, where concrete, one-family homes leak water from the ceilings, whether it's raining or not.

Doña María greeted me as if she'd known me all my life. First, we planted the pine tree, then she squirreled away the cacao, offered me some coffee, and we sat down to a talk which rambled on for hours. Here's a short excerpt of our exchange, which was interrupted by several side conversations, a photo album session, and a wonderful supper delivered by a neighbor.

María: A lifetime is a long time. I'm 88 years old, and I've almost always worked as an empirical midwife. I caught my first baby when I was 13, but I didn't keep on working at that time. When I was 18, I married a 40 year-old man. That's when it really began. I had 17 children, and I had them all by myself.

M: No one helped you to give birth?

María: No one. No one ever helped me, nor has anyone seen my private parts. I've never been admitted to a hospital. When I felt the pains coming, the old man would go into town to shop or do other errands; then I would put wood on the stove and give birth alone. It wasn't easy, but I did what I had to do. Seventeen children.

M: What position did you get into to give birth so many times?

María: Come into my room, and I'll show you. When I felt the labor pains, I got on my knees and held on to the bedpost here, shaking my belly all the while.

M: Is that the position you have other women get into to give birth?

María: No, I have them lie down on their backs. That's how they like to do it.

M: Can you describe your work as a midwife?

María: Let's say you're my client, and you've come for my help. If you've never given birth before, the first thing I do is check to see if you're wide enough for a baby to come out of you. If I see that you're not, I'll tell you, "When you feel the first labor pains, go straight to the hospital so that they'll be able to do a Caesarean on you."

I also check your belly to see if the child is positioned to come out head-first or by its bottom, in a breech position.

M: And if it's coming out breech?

María: Then I rub and rub and rub and rub your belly. If the baby's little head is here on top, I massage you so that it ends up down here at the bottom.

Let's say you come to me four months pregnant, and I see that you're going to have twins. I'll prepare you so that they'll both come out head first, just right.

My granddaughter recently came when she was four months along in her pregnancy for one of my massages. The baby was upside down, but I didn't say anything to her about it. I just told her to stop by every once in a while so I could massage her. When she was ready to deliver, I put three sheets and two pillows on the floor, she lay down, and the baby came out perfect.

M: What if I haven't come to see you so soon in my pregnancy? What if I am nine months pregnant, and the baby is in a breech position?

María: I'd tell you to go to the doctor, because I can't change a baby's position so late in the pregnancy. For that, I have to see you during the fourth month.

I'm going to tell you something. . . . I can tell by the color of the mother's nipples, if the child will be a boy or a girl.

M: How did you learn all this?

María: After giving birth to 17 children all by myself? I guess I should know something about it.

Listen, my first child was born when I'd only been married eight months. He was a seven monther. So I know, when they tell me that a child weighing four or five pounds or more has been in the making for only seven months. No one can fool me. And I'll tell you something else, I've never performed any of those dirty operations. Never, never, never. I'm not that kind of woman.

M: Have you had good luck with the babies you've helped to deliver?

María: Honey, I've never lost a mother, and my only stillborn child was a poor little thing with two heads. No other child has died in childbirth with me.

M: And more or less how many births have you attended?

María: Don't ask me that. One of my daughters has six children, but that's nothing. All the others have 10, up to 16. And that's just my own family! How many births have I attended? I could never count them. I've been working for so many years, and working constantly. Children are born easily with me, thank God.

Once my daughter said she wanted to give birth in town, although she'd already had four with me at home, with no complications at all. I told her, "If you want to go to town, let's go." So we went into town with her husband and all, and as soon as we got her to the hospital, she gave birth. There was no need for her to be hospitalized, but she was. All the nurses asked me, "What happened to you, doña María?," so I had to explain that my daughter had wanted to give birth in town. But her husband said, "Listen, from here on in, no child of mine is going to be born in town!" (laughter)

She had more after that.

M: At home, I guess.

María: Yes. It's much, much better at home.

Thanks to God and the Virgin Mary, I've never had any real problems with the births I've helped along. Nowadays women get pregnant and they go to the hospital and the hospital gives them milk. But it's a cold kind of milk! And they walk around all day, up and down with store-bought milk so that their babies can drink out of bottles. Well, I'd never give that to my own. I brought my children up on breast milk. I never gave them a bottle, never in my life. Never, never, never. And now, so much of that junk.

M: Today, even in the United States, where so much of that store-bought milk is manufactured, doctors recognize that breast milk protects the baby from infection and disease. I've also heard that the muscle tone in the mouths of children who breast feed is much better than those who nurse from bottles. Breast feeding is pretty common in the U.S. now.

María: I should hope so.

M: So let's say that I've come to you because I'm in labor. I'm going to give birth now. What will you do?

María: I'll stay here with you. Every time you have a pain, I'll give you a rub with a special ointment and a strong tea of anise (*anís*) seeds with the leaves of coffee senna (*hedionda chiquita*). That tea helps to eliminate gas, and if there's pain, it relieves the pain, as well.

But maybe you're not pregnant, love. Maybe you've come for a special massage because your leg or foot is injured or out of place. I make those kinds of adjustments, too. I rub the area with a special alcoholated lotion (*alcoholado*) infused with plants .

M: Like bay rum?

María: Bay rum and other plants, including nutmeg. Love, if you have a terrible headache or fever, you can just rub yourself a little with my lotion, and your headache will disappear.

Maybe you've come with a really bad leg and I begin to massage it with alcoholated rubs. I'll be able to tell if it is really broken or just out of joint, and I'll make the adjustments you need, little by little.

M: What if someone has a terrible pain in the kidneys? What do you do then?

María: I rub with something warming like udder balm, and later I do a *santigüo* massage-blessing in the sign of a cross.

M: How did you learn to give that kind of blessing?

María: I learned from Leo Negrón's father, in Pelleja, where I grew up. He taught me instead of teaching his own son, when we were youngsters. The truth is, you can only teach three people during your entire lifetime.

M: Have you already taught your three people?

María: Of course, many years ago. I can't teach you or anyone else now.

M: But you're still helping people with those massages of yours. . .

María: Yes, when someone's leg is badly injured or when someone falls and breaks an arm, I fix them up. And I've never left anyone lame or disabled. Not one person in all my years!

M: I see a few medicinal plants here in your garden.

María: I've always used geranium (*geranio*) tea for flu, and the broadleaf coriander (*recao*) in my garden is good with garlic (*ajo*), onion, and sweet pepper as a base (*sofrito*) for cooking just about everything.

M: Do you have any home remedies that aren't made from plants?

María: I have a remedy that will break anyone of the rum-drinking habit. First you have to catch a dozen *fliches*, those insects that jump on the top of the water. Toast them a bit in a pot so that they get a bit reddish, and leave them for eight days in a bottle of rum. Later you strain the contents of that bottle into an empty one and you make a gift of that bottle to the person with the drinking problem. Well, that person will get a tremendous case of diarrhea and nausea, but s/he'll thank you for it because s/he'll never touch rum again. I tried it on my granddaughter, and she's never had another drink. Yes, she left that habit behind for the rest of her life, and it's a good thing, because if she'd continued she'd be dead by now. Her husband even left her because of her drinking. But now she's married again, and she doesn't touch the stuff. (laughter)

We sit on the front porch of her home as she rolls a thick, loose cigar of fresh-dried tobacco.

María: I buy a yard of tobacco for a dollar, and I roll my own cigars.

M: It smells strong.

María: That's how I like it, strong. Try it.

M: Not bad, and I bet it's good for the circulation. I feel my whole body heating up.

María: Naturally.

We sit silently smoking.

M: I noticed when I went into your room before that you light a lot of candles. Would you tell me something about your spiritual practice?

María: I give all the money I receive for my work to the Catholic church, and they bring me communion three times a month. And yes, my girl, I light candles every single night, to pray with. The candles are for the Virgin Mary, for the saints, for the dead, for the souls. If you're my friend and you die, I light a candle for your soul. And I never sleep until the candles go out. Sometimes I light five or six, sometimes more. Because at times, the dead have the greatest need.

M: Doña Maria, it's been such an honor to talk with you. . . .

María: You know, I never went to school, and I never learned to read or write. Not a word.

M: But you offer a tremendous service to all the people who need you.

María: That's true. Everyone knows me, and they all come to see me. People from the bank, from the drug store, even the police. Once a policeman came here to get a healing rub, but he took off his police jacket before he came inside. He knew I could help him, but he didn't want anyone else to see him coming here to my place. Imagine that (laughter). Just imagine!

Herb Women of Mayagüez

Brunilda Vargas Muñiz and
Primi Socorro Vargas

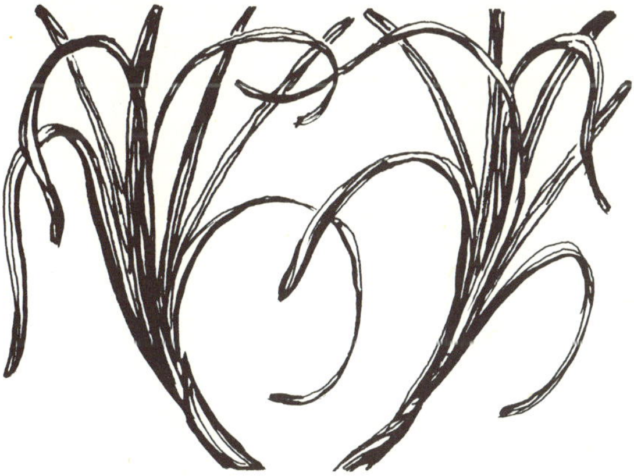

lemon grass *el limoncillo*

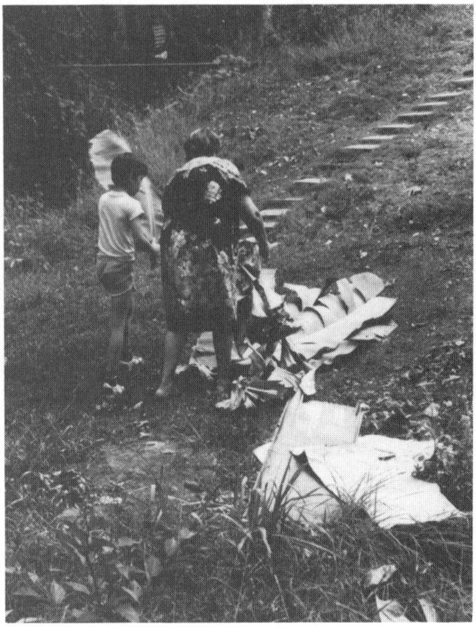

Brunilda and grandson Victor

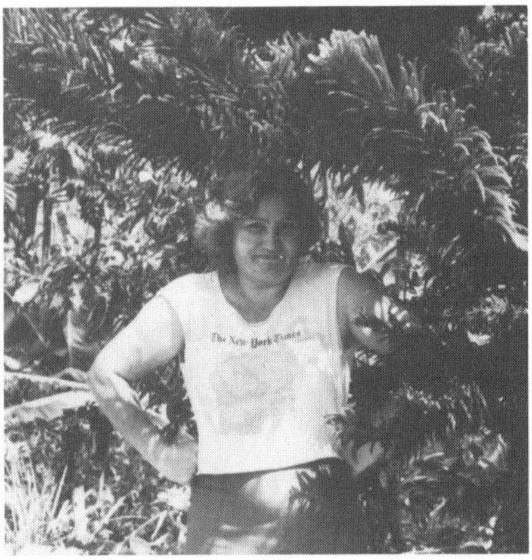

Primi Socorro Vargas

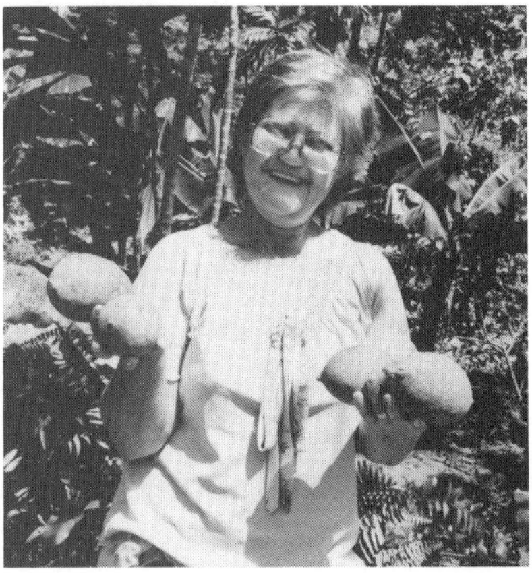

Brígida with jagua fruit

Herb Women of Mayagüez

Brunilda Vargas Muñiz and Primi Socorro Vargas

Brunilda Vargas Muñiz and Primi Socorro Vargas live in the outskirts of Mayagüez on adjoining plots of land that yields fat plantains, bananas, mangos galore, native lentils, medicinal herbs, and a good assortment of *viandas*. Bruni, grandmother of two, works in town as cooking supervisor at a community program for senior citizens. There, because of her knowledge of medicinal plants, she is affectionately known as "*la yerbetera*," the herb woman. Primi Socorro is a licensed beautician with a remarkable memory for the traditions passed on to her from her grandparents.

Both women are proud of their heritage, and knowledgeable about traditional agriculture and healing. Inventive and resourceful, they know how to make do with little, and their generosity abounds. Besides teaching me about the plants on their land, they helped me to organize a book of pressed plants, and taught me to cook from scratch (that means chopping down and smoking the banana leaves too!) the most exquisite *pasteles* I have ever tasted, plus *arroz con dulce*, and *dulce de coco* on an old fashioned wood fire seasoned with lots of earthy humor.

Bruni: I was born in 1929, and I'm proud to say that I grew up in the countryside of Puerto Rico, land of yucca, the singing *coquí*, and everything that's good to eat.

There were seven kids in the family, and we all worked the land and harvested breadfruit (*pana*), sugar cane (*caña*), *jobos*, guava fruit (*guayaba*), tamarind (*tamarindo*), bananas (*guineo*), and much more. We kids were responsible for feeding the animals and carrying water to them in big buckets from the stream. We had pigs, cows, chickens, roosters, rabbits, goats, and more, so after school we had lots of work to do. I made it to the eighth grade.

If we were stung or bitten by an insect, we would crush some garlic and put it on the bite so that it wouldn't swell up. If we got cut, we chopped up a leaf of *sueldaconsuelda*, mixed it with cooking oil, and stuck it on the wound as a poultice. That helped it to heal quickly.

For muscle aches, we used baths of mugwort (*altamisa*), *higuillo oloroso, vara prieta, tártago*, and bay rum (*malagueta*). You always felt like new after one of those baths.

If a woman was about to give birth, we offered her nutmeg (*nemoscá*) tea and bandages soaked in analgesic ointments like "belladonna" and *triaca* "ointment of the air" for the pain. After the birth, she had to drink lots of chicken broth with burnt bread.

For ringworm, we used squash resins mixed in equal parts with the crushed leaves of the ringworm tree (*talantro*).

Arrowroot (*maranta*) was a favorite with every mother because, dried and grated fine, it made an excellent powder for burns and skin eruptions, especially for children. It even helped women who were temporarily sterile because of what we used to call "congested tubes." Those women would boil up the grated arrowroot tubers, mash them into gruel, and eat it by the tablespoonfuls. We had remedies for everything.

And of course, we all enjoyed making bowls for washing rice and shelling gandules, cups for drinking coffee, and serving spoons from gourds of the *higüera* tree.

For all of these reasons and many many more, I'm proud of my Puerto Rico. I learned how to be a real *campesina* here, and that's what I'll be for as long as I live.

M: Can you talk about the land that you live on now?

Bruni: I was born and raised here, and I've never roamed any further than San Juan, because Puerto Rico is my home, and I like it. I inherited this piece of land from my father, and I love to grow native lentils (*gandules*), yams (*ñame*), you name it. I plant every kind of seed that finds its way into my hands, and I have good luck with the plants.

Lately I've been planting a lot of medicinal herbs: red mint (*yerba buena*), lemon balm (*toronjil*), *malá blanca*, a little bit of everything; but it's been very dry this year, and the chlorinated water that's piped in cuts into the plants; then the ants come, and they're done for. So my harvest is small.

M: How did you learn about medicinal plants?

Bruni: My mother loved to make medicinal teas (*guarapos*). She made a tea for everything.

M: How is a traditional *guarapo* made?

Bruni: First you take about a handful of the root or leaf or flower of the plant or plants you need. Then you wash it all very well. When it's clean, you add it all to a few cups of boiling water, lower the flame and cover it. After ten or fifteen minutes of simmering, the water will turn deep green. When it has a good color, you turn off the flame and let it cool. All *guarapos* should be drunk a bit warm in the evening; during the day they can be taken cold, like water, without sugar or anything else.

M: Was making *guarapos* your mother's specialty?

Bruni: My mother could prepare just about anything. She used to make lots of *menorativas*, medicinal *guarapos* using seven, eight, up to ten or more different herbs. Usually, these mixtures are used to help clear out the lungs and bronchial passages.

I'm going to tell you a story, not because I'm proud of myself, but because I'm proud of the tradition handed down to me from my mother. They were always saying to her, "Make me a *guarapo*," and she always would. Well, I'm the same way, and at work they call me "*la yerbetera*," the herb woman.

The other day, my director at work said, "Hey Bruni, my mother's really sick."

She had a flu and a really bad cough along with it, so I took a small handful of *cohitre blanco*, a chopped up "leaf" of spineless (*tuna*) cactus, some red mint leaves (*yerba buena*) and chamomile (*manzanilla*) flowers, a small handful of *paletaria*, two juicy aloe vera (*sábila*) leaves, and finally, a small handful of white basil (*albahaca blanca*) because it's very good for chest colds. Then I washed everything and cooked it up all together, covered, for about twenty minutes in two litres of water.

M: Where did you get that recipe?

Bruni: I learned it from my mother. I haven't forgotten a thing she taught me. And the next day, my director came up to me and said, "Congratulations, Bruni. Mommy was really suffering before she took that remedy you made her. She had a terrible fever with asthmatic attacks, but she's feeling good now."

Her mother also called to thank me, saying that before she

took the remedy she could hardly breathe; she actually thought she'd have to be hospitalized. "I took two cups with honey," she said, "and I began to feel better right away."

Then, when I went to work the next week, my director said, "You have to make me more of that remedy. Last week's supply is all gone."

So I made this one a little stronger. I added some ginger (*jengibre dulce*) and some *poleo* for the cough and hoarseness, and she was very happy with the recipe. Now she feels totally cured!

M: Do you know of a simpler remedy for a bad cold?

Bruni: For a bad cold with fever, the simplest and best thing is a *guarapo* of *gran señora*, which is extremely bitter. Like *botón de cadete*, it will always cut a fever. Later in the garden, I'll show you some lemon grass (*limoncillo*), which also cuts fevers. Lemon grass is delicious too, and blends well with the more bitter herbs.

M: What about the elderly people you work with? Do you ever get a chance to try your remedies out on them?

Bruni: I use one plant for almost all of their digestive complaints. A tea of Caribbean vervain (*verbena*) with lemon seems to do them good no matter what problems they may have, from chronic stomach ache to diarrhea. And it grows right there on the patio.

M: Besides *guarapos* and *menorativas*, what are some other ways of using herbs?

Bruni: In baths, I use aromatic plants and others, like *campana* and *vara prieta* which are normally not taken as beverages. Actually, *vara prieta* can be taken internally, but only for parasites.

For a healing bath, you first get all soaped up, and you use the bath water you've prepared to rinse the soap off your entire body. After letting the bath water run over the body, you wrap the person up in warm clothes and blankets so that he or she can sweat a lot; the very process of sweating helps to eliminate the illness. I learned that from my parents.

We also use plants directly on the skin as poultices. Whenever people got cut badly, they'd go to see my mother because she had *malá* plants, which stop the bleeding. She had a lot of godchildren, whose mothers loved and respected her alot. They'd say, "Go see your godmother. She has *malá*." First, Mom would mash up the stalks of the plant and tie them on to the cut. Once the bleeding stopped, she would apply another medicine, like Humphreys Udder Balm, or belladonna ointment. By the way, belladonna ointment is also great for headaches. Or she would use the gas we used to have in the old days.

M: You mean kerosene?

Bruni: Could be, but we called it gas, and we used it in our lanterns. After letting the lantern burn during the evening, we would simply drip the cool, burned "gas" into the open flesh, and it would cure cuts and wounds of any size. We used it a lot for the animals especially, because besides speeding up the healing process, it kept flies out of the wounds.

We also used the spineless tuna cactus, which makes a wonderful, cooling poultice especially for muscular aches and pains of the lower back and kidneys. You just slice it lengthwise and place it flat on your back, with the wet side on your skin. If you have internal bleeding or an internal infection, what we call *tabardillo*, it's good to cook up one big "leaf" of the tuna cactus with a handful of raw corn in a litre of water and then drink it, as if it were regular drinking water or juice. It's very medicinal.

M: Did you ever use beef tallow (*sebo de Flandes*) as medicine?

Bruni: Not medicinally, but we did use it when our shoes were too tight. My father used to go into town to buy us shoes, but he just guessed our sizes. When he got home, we each took the shoes that fit us best. We really needed that *sebo de Flandes* to keep from getting blisters and callouses.

M: Many women I know suffer from infections of the reproductive system. Up north, we use antiseptic herbs, from garlic to myrrh and goldenseal as internal washes. Here in Puerto Rico, how do you treat that kind of infection?

Bruni: I don't know about serious infections, but for menstrual difficulties, we always prepared a *guarapo* of chamomile, because although it is not quite hot, it is a warming herb. Most often, we'd mix it with red mint and black nightshade (*mata gallina*). To that decoction, add some well washed and chopped-up tuna cactus, which is cooling, and take it as a beverage throughout the day as if it were water.

M: I've heard a little about the theory of heating and cooling plants here in Puerto Rico, and you've mentioned that tuna cactus is cooling, while chamomile has warming qualities. Can you talk more about that?

Bruni: There are cooling plants which are basically refreshing, like mallow (*malva*), tuna cactus, red mint (*yerba buena*), lemon balm (*toronjil*), *paletaria*, mint (*menta*), black nightshade, and *cohitre blanco*. They are all really good for when you have a condition of heat, in the stomach, for instance.

M: And the heating herbs?

Bruni: Some of the hot herbs are *poleo*, ginger (*jengibre*), *gran señora, botón de cadete*. And aloe vera (*sábila*) is heating. If you cut open a stalk of it and add some of its liquid to a tea and serve it, you'll see how warming it is. It's good for chest pains if you ever have a bad cold with a cough.

Chamomile (*manzanilla*), which is basically warm, is also very effective for mixed conditions. You might have a fever within, while feeling cold on the outside; or you may feel cool, but unable to eat, a symptom of overheating. That's when chamomile is especially good, along with something cooling like *cohitre blanco*. That way, the remedy corresponds with both the heat and cold of the condition.

M: What about broken bones and dislocated joints? How did you treat that sort of condition?

Bruni: Now it's a plaster cast, but most often in those cases, my mother gave alcohol or ammonia rubs so that the joints would remain supple and easy to move later on. She made bandages out of fabric soaked in the same liquids. When a finger was twisted or swollen, we gave it pretty much the same treatment.

My mother's heating rubs were very important because we almost never wore shoes, except to go into town, and the soles of our feet would get pretty darn cold.

One of the heating liquids she used to rub us with was called *Aguarrás*. It was also good for getting rid of fleas, lice, ticks and other pests from the house. She used to mix it with undiluted ammonia solution and mop the house with it. It worked!

M: I've heard some people mention using ammonia solution for toothaches. How did you treat that type of problem?

Bruni: If the toothache was really bad, we might actually pull the tooth.

M: Didn't it bleed terribly, then?

Bruni: If it did, my mother would simply say, "Go to the kitchen and bring me two grains of salt," because in those days, salt came in grains. That salt was crushed up and placed where the tooth had been, without rinsing for a while. Salt cleanses and also cuts the bleeding fast.

M: But doesn't it burn?

Bruni: At first it burns a little in the open wound, but you can take it for a while, and then it stops hurting.

If it's hemorrhaging, you can use *salvia* leaf buds. You simply wash, chew, and hold them in place on the gum itself. In a short time the blood coagulates and the pain stops.

M: Bruni, perhaps you can talk about your own experience as a grandmother. What herbs and natural medicines do you use most often at home these days?

Bruni: Nowadays, very few people believe in what grandmothers and grandfathers know. My daughter always tells me, "I'm going to the hospital." And I tell her, "Well, if you really don't want to try one of my home remedies, you don't have to." That's the way it is with my grandchildren, so what are you going to do?

But I use a great deal of witch hazel solution (*Agua Maravilla*) myself. It says here on the label that you shouldn't drink it, but I add it to several preparations. I added two tablespoons along with some honey to the two-litre *menorativa* I made for my director's mother, after I had boiled the whole thing up. Witch hazel solution is used a great deal for colds when there's a lot of phlegm in the chest.

M: That's probably because the witch hazel plant is very astringent. Up north, midwives use the bark of witch hazel to stop hemorrhaging as well.

Bruni: I've never seen that plant, but if we go out into the garden we'll get to look at some of the plants that are growing here right now.

In the following portion of the interview, we are joined by Primi Socorro Vargas y Brígida Sotomayor Vargas, roosters, dogs, children, and the enticing smells of crushed leaves, stems and roots. Surrounded by an atmosphere of joyful noise, fresh air, and good humor, Primi Socorro introduces herself:

Primi: I was the first of eight children born of humble parents in 1944. My father was a farmer; my mother, a seamstress; but I grew up with my grandparents.

My grandfather loved to work the land. He really enjoyed harvesting sugar cane (*caña*), coffee (*café*), yams (*ñames*), oranges (*chinas*), plantains (*plátanos*), and all the island products we love. My grandmother enjoyed planting fruit trees and medicinal plants. For every illness or accident, she had a home remedy growing right in her garden.

I grew up in the countryside, and from the time I was three years old, I ran around the mountains chasing after the chickens, cows and pigs, eating mangos, bananas and oranges off the trees. As I grew up I learned to love and cultivate the land; I also learned home remedies for all kinds of conditions.

For instance, we wrapped bumps and bruises with rags soaked in cold salt water. If the skin swelled and blackened without going down after two or three days, we would use rags soaked with very hot salt water to break up the coagulated blood and bring down the swelling. If you had a bloody wound, perhaps from stepping on a nail, we would apply wood ashes mixed with roasted and well ground, dry coffee, wrapped up in rags.

And coffee was also good if someone had a migraine. First, we would heat up enough *salvia* leaves to cover the entire forehead and temples. Then we'd add a paste of roasted coffee and cooking oil on top of the leaves, place them on your head and wrap them all up with a towel. After lying down for a few hours with that bandage tied on to your head, you felt tremendous relief.

Bruni: Look here. For diabetes, you can take *guarapos* of native lentil (*gandul*) leaf buds or almond leaves. You just drink that tea as if you were drinking water, cold from the refrigerator during the day, warmed up at night.

M: Are you saying that if I have diabetes, drinking these teas will cure me so that I can eat whatever I want?

Bruni: No, but if you drink these teas instead of soda and juice, you'll see that when you go to the doctor the level of sugar in your blood will have gone down quite a bit. And your doctor will suggest that you keep drinking them.

Primi: Look, this is *paletaria*; it's very cooling. When you have a stomach ache, you take a *guarapo* of *paletaria* and your discomfort simply vanishes.

And here is *gran señora*. It's one plant that really dries a condition up. My grandmother used to make me teas of *gran señora* when we had a cold with fever.

M: (I taste *gran señora*.) Holy cow! That's the bitterest plant I've ever tasted. Ahhhhrgh. It's almost unbearable!

Bruni: It's very bitter, and while a guarapo of *gran señora* lowers fever, it's really a powerful heating plant.

Here we have red mint which, mixed with chamomile, is very good for stomach aches. You can always add *paletaria*, too.

ched poison ivy. We just chew up the leaves, and apply that green mass directly as a poultice. If the problem is on a small area of the body, like a finger or toe, you can even use a whole leaf to tie the little poultice on. It's a sort of universal bandage!

Brígida: And they say that it's effective taken in the form of *guarapo*, even in cases of cancer!

M: Would you say that common plantain is a cooling plant or a heating one?

Bruni: It has qualities of both. It cuts pain and it cuts fever, something like chamomile.

Here we have a sour orange tree (*el naranjo*). The leaves are good boiled up in *guarapo* for a chest cold . . .

Brígida: And for upsets. When you need to calm down, they're tranquilizing.

Primi: Not only that, but the same leaves give a wonderful flavor to food. And orange leaves are great in tea, just for fun, especially with honey or sugar.

Here's rue (*ruda*), which is very good for women's pains and problems.

M: I've read that in large quantities it can cause abortion, but most women I've talked with use it in small doses for menstrual discomfort.

Bruni: That's right. And this is *bruja*, which is good for earaches. You warm up the leaf, then crush it and soak up the juice with a little piece of cotton. Then you put the piece of cotton in your ear while it's still warm, and as the liquid from the cotton seeps out into the ear, the pain goes away.

M: What is this little tree good for?

Bruni: It's *tártago*, good for all sorts of enchantments. (laughter)

Brígida: People who work with the spirit world often plant these trees in front of their homes.

Primi: But not only that. See this resin? It can be used to get rid of callouses and corns. Rub the sap on the callous with a little piece of cotton.

Bruni: Yes, and when kids want to play with bubbles, here they are! (she blows some of the *tártago* sap off the end of a pine needle, and soap-like bubbles begin to surround her along with lots of laughter.) *Now* you're learning something useful here!

Primi: Here we have *vara prieta* which, along with *cariaquillo* and mango leaves, make a bath to remove all negative energies. Plants like *sacabuche* and *Santa María* are also used. Basically, it's a psychological thing. The herb woman prescribes this kind of warm bath, and people feel beter. It could have something to do with the faith they have . . . in the plants and also in the *yerbetera*.

Bruni: The same bath is also good for muscle aches and rheumatism.

M: Up north, we have plants that are like soap; they foam and remove dirt to some extent. Do you have any soapy plants like that here?

Bruni: When someone has dandruff, we apply aloe vera as if it were shampoo, just the juice as it comes out of the stem, raw.

Primi: And if your child happens to have head lice, you can boil up the vines of *cundeamor* until the water turns green; then you use it as if it were a shampoo, but leave it on the kid's head for a good 15 or 20 minutes afterwards. That kills the lice; it's good for the scalp. And remember, you're talking with a beautician. I know!

M: As a beautician, can you talk about some of the plants you use for cosmetic purposes?

Primi: Avocado makes a good head massage for dry hair, and it's excellent for dry skin. You can just rub it into the scalp or the skin and leave it for about twenty minutes or so.

I also use coconut oil when people start losing their hair. Rub it in and give a good massage with it daily; it really stimulates the scalp.

And coconut water is the best thing for the kidneys; it's very soothing. So is "closed" monkey's hand (*baquiña cerrada*). It has a round leaf, and it's excellent for treating kidney stones.

Brígida: *Juana la blanca* is also used in tea for kidney stones but I've heard that it's dangerous to use on a long-term basis. It supposedly damages the liver.

Primi: All I know is that it gives you lots of gas!

Bruni: Here we have amaranth (*blero*), another cooling herb. It makes a good tea for heating conditions, especially for the kidneys, when there is infection. Served cold, it's quite refreshing, and similar to *cohitre blanco* in its effect.

M: It tastes like a kitchen vegetable.

Bruni: Of course; it *is* a vegetable, something like purslane (*verdolaga*). All three are cooling, and that's how they heal.

M: In New York, cream of purslane soup is considered a real delicacy, and it's also quite popular in salads.

Primi: It makes a calming, nourishing tea, too.

M: That's good to know because I like to drink nourishing teas every day.

Primi: Well, the refreshing herbs we've mentioned: *cohitre blanco,* amaranth, purslane, *paletaria*, and black nightshade (*mata gallina*) would all be perfect. Now, if you want to stimulate the circulation, you might try ginger tea. It's really warming.

Bruni: Here's annato (*achiote*), which is good for circulation. We use the leaves for hot baths when someone has muscle spasms. It really helps. And the seeds themselves are used for giving color to food, especially to *pasteles**.

Primi: Here is *santa María*, which is also used in baths. It's one of the plants that goes into making a type of *Agua Florida* (a popular alcohol rub).

And here is *campana*, which is used primarily for baths. Lately though, people have used it as a drug to make them dopey. It makes you feel slow and stupid.

Bruni: Some young people have actually been brain damaged from using it. It's a terrible waste. But as medicine, the plant has always been useful, especially for women.

M: Have you ever used valerian (*valeriana*)?

Primi: Of course, for my nerves. When I was little, I was always so nervous, but my grandmother brought me some valerian root, and after taking just three *guarapos*, I was just fine. It was the blessed cure!

M: Maybe you got cured fast because you just couldn't bear the taste! (laughter) I usually prepare valerian in alcohol as a tincture so that I can use just a small amount because it has such a strong smell and flavor.

Primi: I didn't mind the flavor at all. I drank it right down, without sugar or any sweetener, even. That's the best way to get to know your plants, after all.

Bruni: This flower here is called the fairy rose (*rosa cienhojas*). It makes a very good eyewash for conjunctivitis. Just leave half a dozen of the roses in water overnight, and use the water to rinse the eyes with throughout the next day.

Primi: Look, that's mallow (*malva*), another cooling plant. It makes a great tea for the kidneys, and when your skin erupts in boils or little cysts, it's an excellent poultice. Just wash the area with the water you've boiled the leaf in, then place the boiled leaf on top of the cyst. Drink the water, even! Malva water douches are also good for inflammations of the uterus.

And *tuatúa* is another great plant for cysts or boils. If you have an external cyst that isn't opening up, you can put a heated leaf of *tuatúa* on top of it, and leave it there until it bursts open. I'm speaking from experience. That's how I got rid of a tumor the size of a hen's egg. And what a place to have it! I saw stars everytime I sat down.

M: How did you use it?

Primi: I remember it as if it were yesterday, but actually, it was years ago on New Year's Eve. The only way I could bear the pain was to spread my legs so far apart that one was heading for Maricao and the other for San Germán*. My grandfather had just died a little while before that, and I prayed to him, asking him to illuminate my mind. "What can I do to make this cyst go away?" I asked him. Then I got the idea of using *tuatúa*, and Bruni went and got some for me. First I boiled up some leaves and while that water was cooling down a bit, I warmed and softened up another leaf by passing it back and forth over a low flame. Then I washed the area with the warm "tea," and put the warm leaf on the cyst, covered with a little oil in order to keep it stuck to my skin. The idea is that it's a "drawing" plant; it draws out to the surface whatever is causing the problem inside. Well, just about midnight, the cyst burst open and I got rid of blood, pus, everything that was inside. All the excesses of my system seemed to be located in that one place.

M: How did you deal with the open wound after that?

Primi: I boiled some more *tuatúa* leaves, and with the water left over, I rinsed it well. Finally, I applied some special cream the doctor recommended, but to my mind, the cure came from the *tuatúa*. I'd had the cyst for more than two weeks, and the doctor had said he'd have to operate by January 2 if it hadn't burst by then. Imagine living with the pain of a surgical wound in that place! So at last it did burst open and left only a tiny scar, thanks to God and the Virgin; and I have witnesses!

Bruni: I don't know if you know the *maya* plant. My grandmother used it when she wanted to coagulate milk to make cheese. It has tiny thorns and a little tassel. You add that little fruit to milk, and it sours quickly.

Primi: Of course, lemon coagulates milk too, and it's very good for the skin as well. It cuts right through oil and pimples, plus it helps in the digestion of heavy, greasy foods like shellfish. And lemonade is the most refreshing drink in the world when you're very hot.

Brigida: Not to mention for arthritis. I take it every morning, and it has really helped me a lot.

M: What about home remedies that aren't plants? One of the older women I interviewed mentioned that children's urine could be poured over the forehead of someone with a fever in order to lower the fever. I'd never heard of that remedy outside of the island.

Primi: That's an old fashioned treatment; it also works when you have a cramp in your leg or foot. I've never tried it myself, but my grandmother used it a great deal.

Bruni: She's right; you end up with no cramp at all.

Brígida: There's another remedy for leg cramps. We always rubbed corn silk into the cramped area, and it worked!

Primi: You know, my uncle always used to say that urine could be used if a wasp bit you; it cut the pain.

M: And I know it works for jelly fish bites, maybe because of its ammonia content.

Primi: Raw garlic is also really good for the pain of insect and animal bites, and it's antiseptic.

Brígida: Even the doctors are saying that taken internally, garlic lowers the blood pressure.

There is a silence, suddenly filled with Primi's laughter.

Primi: Look at Bruni chewing breadfruit gum! (laughter)

Bruni: When I was a child following my father around the farm, he'd tell me, "I'm going to go and cut the breadfruit (*pana*) tree so that tomorrow you'll have some chewing gum." And the next morning, I went to the tree and got my chewing gum. You can chew and chew and chew the sap.

M: What does it taste like?

All: Like breadfruit!

Primi: Which reminds me. It's time to cook. Who wants *bacalao con pana?*

Two Espiritistas of Loíza

doña Casimira and doña Bolina

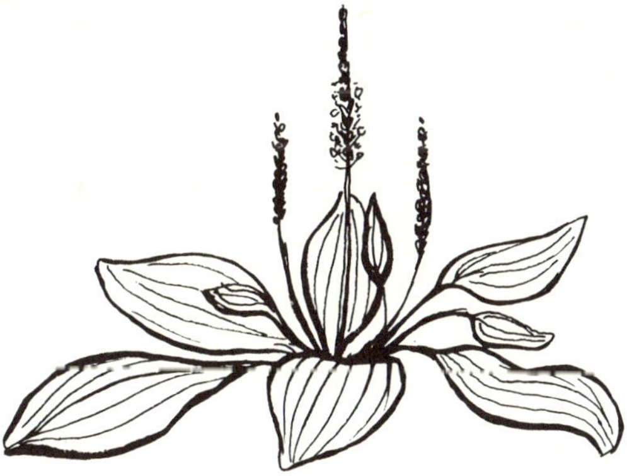

common plantain *el llantén*

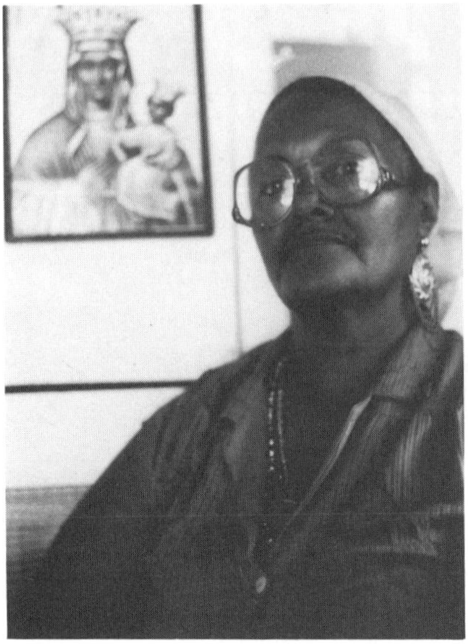

doña Bolina

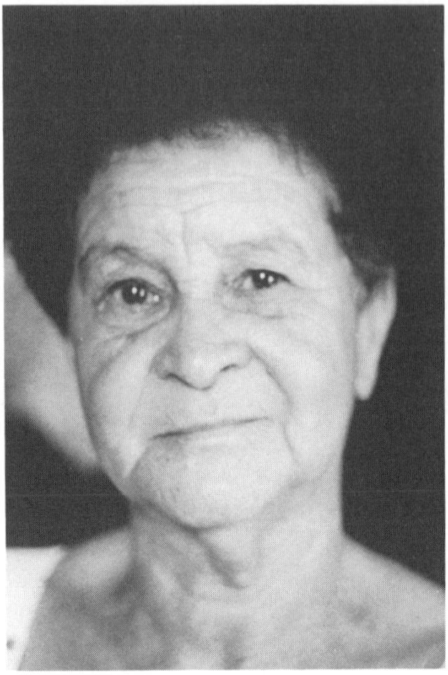

doña Casimira

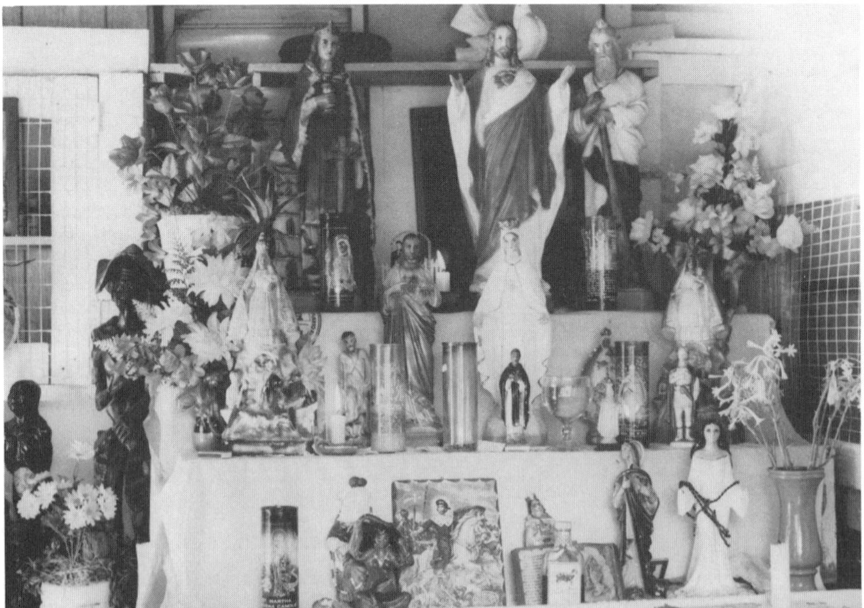

One of doña Bolina's altars

Two Espiritistas of Loíza

doña Casimira and doña Bolina

The village of Loíza Aldea is an important center of Afro-Caribbean culture in Puerto Rico. Like many coastal towns, it supported a thriving sugar cane industry worked mostly by Black slaves for generations. After slavery was abolished, Loíza was home to a large population of free African-Americans who, isolated from the main roads which linked other towns, managed to preserve many purely African traditions.

Interested in medicinal plants, I went to Puerto Rico with the idea of meeting herbal medicine practitioners. And I found that in Loíza, most people who work with herbs to heal physical ailments are also involved in the mystical realm. The following edited interviews with two independent *espiritistas* (diviners and spiritual healers) of Loíza reflect the use of herbs as well as a variety of psycho-spiritual techniques for healing on many levels. Here, the world of plants and physical healing is integrally linked with spiritual renewal. And humanistic psychological counseling takes place in a context that affirms cultural values.

Although doña Bolina's pragmatism contrasts with doña Casimira's approach, both women recognize faith as the source of their inspiration *and* the secret of their success. Both women discovered their calling during childhood through religious visions, and both are especially devoted to two different aspects of the same saint. Casimira works with the Infant of Prague, the Catholic saint of children, while Bolina works with an African expression[1] of the same spirit—Eleggua—the elder yet childlike deity charged with opening the roads.

Both *espiritistas* show a surprising ability to integrate ancient aspects of their tradition with modern perspectives and practices. Doña Bolina is an initiate of the *palo monte—palo mayombé*[2] tradition. She uses books such as Lydia Cabrera's literary and anthropological *El Monte* as a source of botanical information and prayer, and merges healing through faith with a sophisticated psycho-therapeutic outlook. Doña Casimira offers an expansive, ecumenical definition of God, while her allusion to plant symbology reflects the extent to which the ancient "word magic" of African traditions has been integrated into her practice.

Both women use a rich treasury of symbols (ranging from candles to the saints themselves) to represent certain kinds of thought and awareness. For both, the most important symbols recall the basic healing principles of faith, thanksgiving and love.

[1] During slavery, African people were forced to worship Christian saints. Thus their own pantheon of spiritual beings was syncretized with Christian saints according to the symbolism accrued to those saints in devotional works of art. Thus, for instance, Changó—a male deity associated with lightning—became Saint Barbara, whose visual representations always included a bolt of lightning, and so on.

[2] *Palo, palo monte* and *palo mayombé* are words used to describe the religion of the Bantu speaking people of the African Congolese civilization.

Meeting with doña Casimira

I waited in doña Casimira's parlor for about twenty minutes while she counseled a handsome, early thirties-ish lawyer, a long-time client and friend. He stayed to listen to our interview, which was interrupted several times by other clients who came by to leave offerings and other items to be used in doña Casimira's "works" for them in a little house in the back yard. She made it clear that she was well known as an *espiritista* not only on the island but in far away places as well. After listening to her talk about her work, seeing some evidence of her popularity (one client had come from 90 mountainous miles away to see her), and receiving a highly accurate personal reading, I knew I had found a gifted seer.

Casimira: My work is spiritual work. It comes not from study or anything resembling study, but from the spiritual vision which I receive through my thoughts. I also receive information from sources such as Tarot cards and the spiritual circles we *espiritistas* hold in order to call upon the powers of protection. Whatever I get from these activities I then offer to people who come to me. Most are looking for healing or for ways to increase and enhance their abilities.

I'm no doctor, but I can offer relief to people. Most often I work in order to help people with psychological problems, problems within a marriage, let's say. When people need some perspective, I help them to move ahead correctly. Sometimes people reach the point of abusing themselves with drugs or other vices, and I help them to re-orient themselves.

I work with the divine forces, and if someone is on the wrong path, I tell him or her, "Look, with the evidence that I have here, it looks as if the following is going to happen." A few days later, that person comes to me in tears, saying, "What you said would happen really happened!" That's because I receive help from those above. Some time may elapse, but everything the spirits tell me, comes to pass.

M: Besides just talking with and counseling people, what does your work actually involve?

Casimira: It depends upon what images and what information come to me through my thoughts and intuition.

I use plants a great deal, actually. For psychological problems, baths of mugwort (*altamisa*), aloe (*sábila*), Caribbean vervain (*verbena*) and other symbolic plants can help to cast off negative influences. For this kind of work, I suggest specific baths according to need.

If someone comes to me with stomach problems, I'll do a special massage-anointing in the form of a cross on that person's stomach; this *santigüo* is always accompanied by special prayers. I might also offer that person medicinal teas which are specific for the stomach such as red mint (*yerba buena*), leaves of *poleo,* and *guanábana* buds; these teas are traditionally given after a *santigüo*.

I've also dealt a great deal with skin problems, including a case of what had been called "incurable" eczema. That woman came all the way from Caguas to see me. I told her to apply the boiled leaves of yellow *roble* and to use a special soap; she came back within two weeks and her skin looked better than mine looks now.

M: Have you ever used plants to deal with serious, life-threatening health problems?

Casimira: Absolutely. My own son was at the San Jorge Clinic for a kidney operation not too long ago, and while he was there they [the spirits] told me, "He's going to be OK, and you won't have to go back to the hospital; it's just an added expense." And that was the truth. The treatment they wanted to give him cost over $2,000. Meanwhile, I had also received a prescription through my thoughts: common plantain (*llantén*), *baquiña cerrada*, and *Juana la blanca* boiled up together and strained, to be served with a coconut every morning. Well he endured some intense pain, but the stones left his body.

And not too long ago I actually treated a young woman with an advanced cancer. She couldn't have weighed too much more than forty pounds; one look in her eyes, and you knew she was on her way out. Well, I received the means to help her. I recommended she drink the boiled seeds of *cundeamor* with shoots of anamú and leaves of common plantain. Plantain is recognized almost all over the world as a remedy for cancer. Well, with that medicine, she started discharging everything she didn't need right out of her system. Now she's back to work at the food stamps division of Social Services, and she's just gorgeous; plumper and better looking than the two of us combined.

Half the time we just ignore the medicinal plants, but they are a real aid for human health. And in Puerto Rico, the knowledge about using these plants goes back generations, because our grandparents knew how to take care of all kinds of problems.

M: Do you see that people are turning back to the plants today?

Casimira: Yes, my child. I tell the doctors, "I know you don't believe in plants, but little by little you're losing your patients because more and more people are moving toward natural ways of healing." It's just tremendous how many people are going to natural healers for advice these days.

If you have a bad stomach ache, you boil up some mint to drink, and before you know it, you feel fine. Plants themselves are the best, the most effective and beautiful expression of medicine for human beings.

M: Earlier, you mentioned the use of "symbolic plants." Can you explain that term?

Casimira: It's something that comes down to us from our ancestors. I think people all over the world associate certain plants with symbolism. The world of the spirits corresponds with the world of plants, and the world of the mind—the world of words—also has its correspondence in the world of plants. So that mint (*menta*) eases the mind (*mente*); *salvia* helps one to be acquitted (*salve*) when one is on trial. Plantain (*llantén*) is for a person who weeps (*llanto*). That's one source of the symbolism, and there are others. For instance, the saints themselves each have their associations with plants. But we'll talk about that some other time.

M: You said that you never studied in order to learn this type of work. So how *did* you learn about all of this?

Casimira: It all started for me when I got very sick as a child. I was seven years old, and for five days I was unconscious in my bed. It was a time when no one had money for anything. People made 40 cents for a whole day's work! Plants were the only medicine then, because even if you could afford to see a doctor, you could never afford to buy the pills or whatever he might prescribe. Children died of parasitic infestations with their stomachs all swollen; it was a sad life for so many people. Well, my father managed to afford a doctor, who came to the house to see me. But all he could say was, "Make this girl a coffin; she's dying." Then, as I was hovering between life and death, God spoke to me, "Open your eyes; look at me." And I saw the most beautiful handwriting with letters that said, "You aren't going to die now; you will live a long life. I need you to do some important work." So I asked my mother to bring me some milk, which I drank, and the next day I started eating everything they put in front of me.

From then on, I started saying things to my mother like, "Mommy, so and so has a bad fever. They should put camphor compresses on the soles of her feet. She needs a good sweat tonight." Or if someone had diarrhea, I would receive the means to say, "She should be taking teas of basil (*albahaca blanca*) with cashew (*pajuil*) husks and *hicaco* fruit." So it wasn't something I learned from someone else. God gave me the gift when I was seven years old.

That's why my favorite saint is the Infant of Prague; all my life he has come through with miracles for me. He is the patron saint of children, and helps a great deal when a child is sick or has other problems.

Anyway, my parents were uncomfortable with what I was doing, so they sent me to live with my aunts when I was nine. By the time I was twelve, I started working for people, giving advice, telling them what was going to happen to them and which remedies they should take. Every bit of information I received through my mind, through my thoughts, through my visions, I shared with the people who came to me. Then I decided to stop doing that work until I'd married and raised a child. But when my son was twelve, I began working a lot, and word began to spread. They've come all the way from Canada, from the Virgin Islands, and from New York to see me. All by word of mouth.

M: Can you talk about some of the important things you've learned during the years you've been working?

Casimira: I'm 74 years old, so they've been coming for more than 60 years, and in those years I've learned a few things about people, and about God.

I've seen lots of fighting and hostility among the churches here in Puerto Rico: the Pentecostals, the Evangelists, the Catholics. I remember that one day my mother said to me, "So and so can't go to heaven because they didn't offer a mass for him." And I said, "After someone has led a good life, you mean to tell me he can't go to heaven because some other people didn't pray for him?" That's when it became really evident to me that something was wrong. Because I felt, and I knew, that we can only be judged according to the greatest sacrament in life: loving one's fellow human beings and treating them well.

People used to think that Catholicism was the only way to save people. But I say there's only one church, and all the rest are bastards. The church is God, the God who lives in the heart of every human being. If you help your fellow human beings, then you have God. Because there are people who go to church every day, and then go home to live in ways that are inconsistent with the way of God; they betray real love and caring for others.

M: What qualities are most important in a person who wants to heal or otherwise help others?

Casimira: The most important quality and gift of every human being on earth is faith.

In all that you may do, you must name God first; that's how favor is granted. When you open your hands and you have faith in God, God places His hand in yours. If you sincerely call upon God to help you in your work, then every time you put your hand on someone to heal, it will land in just the right spot. It's a way of healing people through faith. Your hands are blessed by God so that you can heal; you use your hands so that the person receiving the healing can be blessed by God.

You can break through serious psychological problems and even someone's being bewitched if you do an anointing in the name of God. It's all faith, my love. Faith makes life happen. If you don't have faith, you can't do anything.

M: So you just lay your hands on the person . . .

Casimira: I simply place my hand on the person to bless her or him; that's one way of doing it. Other times I might do the massage-anointing in the form of a cross. This *santigüo* healing is accompanied by my own secret prayers. These prayers help with everything. If your head is all blocked up with negative thoughts or with other psychological problems, my hands on your temples and our silent prayers will open things up.

I also find that people need spiritual baths to cleanse themselves of negative energies and take in purity once again. When you are loaded down with problems, you're carrying around an atmosphere or aura that's been tainted. Certain types of baths will help you cleanse yourself and relax.

Every type of bath is different. For luck, you bathe in basil, red mint, and marjoram. Baths to counteract or offset spiritual problems or even manipulation by others may include *poleo*, wormseed (*pazote*) and *salvia*.

M: Can you describe how a spiritual bath is prepared?

Casimira: First you have to boil the plants you'll be using, and let that water cool. Then after bathing yourself with soap and water, you let the plant bath flow over you from your head to your toes, over every part of your body. Then, without drying yourself off, you get out of the tub. You can't sit in the water, because the water has taken with it all the negativity that you don't want or need any longer.

There are baths for everything from muscle aches and arthritis to a broken heart. One thing all of the baths have in common is that they leave you feeling completely pure, and open to purity in your environment.

M: Is there something more you'd like to say to people about what you've learned over the years you've spent working as a healer and spiritual guide?

Casimira: Right now, the entire cosmos is overcharged with an atmosphere of great difficulty; it's an especially rough time for the world, and it demands that people orient themselves through prayer, giving thanks and also asking for positive visions of what might happen.

The most important thing is to pray that you receive ways of working through this era. If you do this, you will then receive visions that will help you.

It is also very important that you live in a grateful way, always carrying with you a symbol of thanks in your thoughts. Those thanks, and your prayers, can break through any bitterness, any heaviness, any difficulty.

It all boils down to prayer, of sincerely searching for God, who offers shelter, grace, and power. Without God, the leaves on the trees do not flutter, because God is nature. And nature is God, in every plant, in every flower, and in every positive thought. God is not present in negative thoughts.

It makes me angry when I hear people say, "Such and such a thing is going to happen, and how horrible!" I always respond by saying, "What's the matter with you? Don't you have any faith?" Because if you do have faith, you will receive great blessings.

If you don't take the risk, if you don't shut your eyes and walk forward with faith in search of higher ground, you can not be charged with a real mission in life, and you'll never be prepared for your destiny.

One person comes to be born for one reason, another for another reason; fulfillment comes through the divine thoughts that put you on your path.

Meeting with doña Bolina

When I turned off the main street onto a slim dirt road, I saw low gray clouds billowing from a tiny house. My escort shrugged, "That's the place," and left me about fifeen yards away. Doña Bolina was performing a *sahumerio* or psychic cleansing of her work space with the heady smoke of myrrh and other resins. She seemed glad to see me, and I was deeply moved by the variety and abundance of sacred images in her space. One wall was lined with a three-tiered altar of the mostly white-skinned Catholic Saints (which, through a process of syncretization, have come to represent the African, mostly Yoruba divinities or orishas), flanked by an altar more clearly representative of African orishas. A third altar supported busts of Indian figures, amulets, and other symbols associated with the island's Taino indigenous heritage. "I have them all," she said with pride, "because the Puerto Rican people are of African, Indian and Spanish descent. These are our roots."

Doña Bolina has built up her trade little by little while raising ten children to adulthood and working her way up for 27 years to the post of personnel supervisor at a nearby factory. "I don't have a formal education," she began. "I just went to the eighth grade; but I do have a spiritual preparation. . . ."

Bolina: When I was five or six years old I felt that the spirit world was talking to me, and I would answer. I saw several visions—apparitions of Christ and the Virgin in many forms—but I didn't begin advising people until I was 25. Even before I was initiated as a priestess I recommended treatments, offering people spiritual therapy. I would suggest which saints to pray to, what kinds of baths to take, which plants to use.

Meanwhile, I got married and had 13 children. That was also part of my preparation. I've been through a lot in life.

M: Can you talk about some of the saints which are represented on your altars?

Bolina: I have all these images of saints here because they reflect the essence of the divine beings. I work with God, and these figures represent aspects of God, so I treat them with a great deal of respect.

Working with the saints is a way of helping people make use of one of their greatest resources, their faith, in order to see and believe in their own strengths.

For instance, Saint Jacinto is the spirit of making peace. Saint Martin helps the poor. Elegguá takes many forms; here he is the Infant of Prague, guide and protector of all children. Saint James is the warrior. Saint Martha conquered the dragon, and helps people to be more assertive. She also helps couples who are fighting to keep peace in their home; the woman who prays to Saint Martha brings the saint into her own heart in order to manage with her husband better. Saint Expedito is the patron of business and money. Saint Jude advocates for those confronted with difficult or impossible situations, and is the patron of all lawsuits. La Caridad del Cobre, Oshún, rules the waters that flow. Saint Barbara has two personalities, man and woman. For six months of the year he is Changó, and during the other six months she is Barbara The

African Saint Barbara with the cut on her face aids those of us who are suffering afflictions. Of course, the Indian spirits are represented here; they are the spirits of our ancestral tribes. And my *madama* figure symbolizes the African religions, the spirit of those who dance to the drums, the spirit of those who work in my field of advice and consultations. I carry on with her work, and when there's a service, I play the drum and we dance in a spiritual way just as the Congo people did, and still do.

M: Do you think that everyone has a special relationship with one of the saints?

Bolina: Everyone has a spiritual guide who acts as a sort of an ideal self. If you believe in this guide, you have to listen to it. For example, one day it just occurs to you, "Today I'm going to make a pan of sweet coconut rice." Well, you just don't let yourself get lazy. You don't say, "Forget it; it's too much work." When you hear your guide's voice telling you to do something, you must follow it and never regret it. Life is a chance for us to prepare ourselves on the spiritual and material planes, and our guides help us to do that.

My own special spiritual guide is Elegguá, who protects me and my children. I might pray, "Elegguá, my spirit guide, you who know the roads of life, put my son on the correct path. Great African divinity, protect my son." Then when I see that my prayers have been answered, I will make an offering to Elegguá. Maybe I'll put a dried coconut behind the door, or I may make a little amulet in the shape of one of Elegguá's implements. That symbol will help to develop my awareness of him and his protection, so I feel better in general. These practices clear your mind.

M: I notice quite a few cigars here. What do they mean to you?

Bolina: I smoke the cigars, as tobacco is a gift of the Indians and of Congo people. I honor these people with my tobacco and with my coffee.

M: Can you talk about what your work of advice and consultation actually involves? What methods do you use to help people?

Bolina: First let me say that faith is at the essence of my work. It is the root of all I do. Because it's really people's faith that heals them in the end. Everything I do myself comes through faith, and I have plenty of it.

I see people suffering from anxiety, people with psychological problems. I help them through spiritual means. When they arrive, they see themselves surrounded by the saints, and they see that I am concentrating on this glass of water. For me, the problems of each person are reflected in this glass of water. I receive information from a spiritual source, and in this cup, I see the physical reality.

If you come to see me, you'll also notice that during our consultation, I'll be scribbling on a piece of paper while the images come to me from the other world. My focusing on the water and writing helps the person to calm down, trust me, and concentrate better.

My response will depend upon what the person tells me and whatever other messages I receive about that person's needs in the cup of water. Let's say there is a psychological problem; I might say, "Someone has made a negative suggestion about you and you've accepted that suggestion. That's what's making you so anxious." Or perhaps there's a marital problem. Most likely I can help in that case too. Remember, I've been married for 42 years.

I've come to learn that if one is not relaxed, nothing will turn out right. So I create a relaxing atmosphere, and then I try to recommend that which will help my visitor to relax the most. Maybe that means sending someone off to church to be still and pray; or maybe it will mean prescribing a special bath of soothing herbs like mugwort (*altamisa*) and bitter orange leaves (*hojas de naranjo*). Or I might recommend that my client drink special soothing teas like linden (*tilo*) or chamomile (*manzanilla*) or orange leaves. Maybe I'll suggest a swim in the ocean in order to cleanse the body and soul of all negativity. If someone can't sleep, I'll tell that person to put a pastille of camphor in a glass of water, and to place that under the bed just before turning in for the night.

One thing is certain; these remedies won't hurt anyone, and if a problem is basically psychological, the very act of preparing a remedy with faith may be healing.

M: Do you have a pretty high rate of success?

Bolina: Oh yes. The remedies I offer almost always work. While I prescribe them, I'm affirming always, "Don't worry; God will take this trial away from you. It will pass." And I say it with a total faith and a soothing voice so that they can really feel that passing.

M: What are the most common problems you've seen among people who've come to you for advice?

Bolina: So many people are traumatized by poverty; they always want what they can't have; they want what rich people have, what they see on television. Well, I've raised ten children to adulthood, and each has a degree and a career. But when they were little, if I just had a little flour in the house, that's what we fried up for breakfast. If there was nothing nice to wear, they had to put on whatever there was. No complaints. So I base some of my advice on this way of looking at things, and always, on my faith.

Sometimes people feel so inferior, they think that other people can actually have power over them. They believe that others are out to get them, that others are capable of bewitching them, of bending their wills. They forget to have faith in themselves, in their own path. They should pay more attention to trying to fight for what they want and believe in, and say "I'm going to do this thing." As long as they're not hurting anyone, they should go ahead and do it.

I also see marital problems, and family problems which come about through a lack of communication and understanding. When parents tell me that their children don't pay them any mind, I tell them to talk to their kids about their own lives. Talk with them about love and about sex, about drugs and alcohol. That's a way of opening communication up so there's more understanding within the family. Talking is a form of therapy in itself.

Another major problem I encounter is self-serving gossip that serves to hurt people. That comes about when people get pleasure out of living their neighbors' lives instead of their own.

I always counsel people to stop looking at what others do and what others have and to learn to live with their own lives. To accept their own lives.

M: Do you ever recommend that someone see a doctor or psychiatrist?

Bolina: Absolutely! I often send people to get help from medical professionals. Sometimes women come suffering from physical ailments, including reproductive problems. I send those women to see a doctor; I never prescribe for illness. And when people are too anxious to even listen to me, I send them to a psychologist or psychiatrist. But in most cases, the high price of going to the doctor is prohibitive.

For the most part, people come to me feeling nervous and anxious and leave feeling calm and tranquil. Sometimes people go to the doctors first, and come to me later just to find that they get more relief through the spiritual healing, and through my work with the plants.

M: Can you talk about the ways you use plants for spiritual and physical healing?

Bolina: If you think you have something like bad energy following you around, I recommend that you take a bath of marjoram, red mint (*yerba buena*), Florida water, or mugwort. If you have a chronic physical problem like an allergy, I might have you boil a green papaya and drink the juice, or lots of cooling teas, such as *paletaria*, spineless (*tuna*) cactus, amaranth (*blero*), or purslane (*verdolaga*). Maybe I'll suggest that you eat lots of cooling fruits and vegetables. Then there are other plants like *cundeamor* and *white gandul* which, while they nourish, are strong medicines as well. They can be taken as teas.

If someone has a cold and doesn't want to see a doctor, I'll say, "Boil up some star anise (*anís de estrella*) as a tea, add some honey, and a few drops of lemon. Tomorrow you'll be a lot better." And lemon—so light and so refreshing—is also good for certain types of headache.

For a cold in the body, a forehead wrap of coffee grounds will help—even if you have a migraine.

Now if someone has a bad stomach ache, I'll probably say, "See a doctor," especially if I think it might be an ulcer. But if the doctor can't help, I'll recommend boiling up some black nightshade (*yerba mora*) in milk, either alone or in combination with leaves of common plantain. That should be taken on a regular basis.

If someone has eye trouble and can't see very well, I'll tell that person to mix some plantain leaves (*llantén*) with rue (*ruda*) and wash them well. Then I recommend they be put in a clean glass of water to be left out during the cool dampness of the night (*al sereno*) so that the plant's juices can be infused in that atmosphere. Then, in the morning you get up and wash your eyes with that water, and you feel much better. Of course, I advise that the person see an eye doctor too.

If someone comes with constipation, feeling stuck, I recommend plenty of coconut water with lemon, a remedy which comes directly from our African heritage.

If you feel very weak, I'll recommend that first you go to the doctor. But if the doctor's treatment doesn't help too much, then take a couple of fresh, raw eggs and make yourself a little punch with fresh milk, half an ounce of brandy or rum, and some brown sugar. I believe that it's good for the body to take an ounce of alcohol two or three times a week. A little bit of everything is good.

M: Where did you learn about all of these remedies?

Bolina: I was trained as a priestess in the tradition of *palo monte,* which is a spiritual tradition that includes healing knowledge; and through the years I've tried many, many remedies which are part of the oral tradition here in Puerto Rico. I also use books on medicinal plants to guide me. For instance, Lydia Cabrera records that amaranth (*blero*) is used to refresh and do spiritual cleansings and renewals. It can even be used as a vegetable. Boiled, it helps the body to cleanse itself, and the leaves cooked for poultices are effective against tumors.

M: Do you know of people who have used amaranth successfully to treat tumors?

Bolina: Yes, both as a poultice and as a drink.

M: That's a powerful plant.

Bolina: But the mind is the most powerful thing. Look. This candle burning here can be seen literally as a means of calling someone to come to me through the five senses, the seven thoughts. But it's actually a tool of thought transmission. I light it here at Saint Barbara's feet, and I tell the woman who waits for a call from her husband, "I lit the candle, and today he's going to call you on the phone." Sure enough, because she has that thought, he will call. Later she'll say that the results were my doing, but really, it was the power of her faith and of her thought.

M: Do you accept money for your work?

Bolina: The people who come to see me always leave a few dollars so I can continue with my work, and so I can buy my candles.

Candles don't mean much to most people, but to me, they symbolize that all-important faith and the bringing of light. I place a candle before each saint and that brings light to the spirit. Plus, they are beautiful.

A Humble Medicine of Earth and Spirit

Cruz María Santiago of Morovis

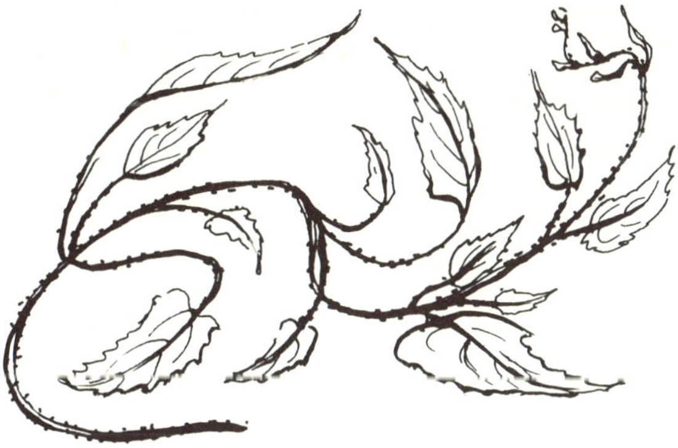

stinging vine *la pringamosa*

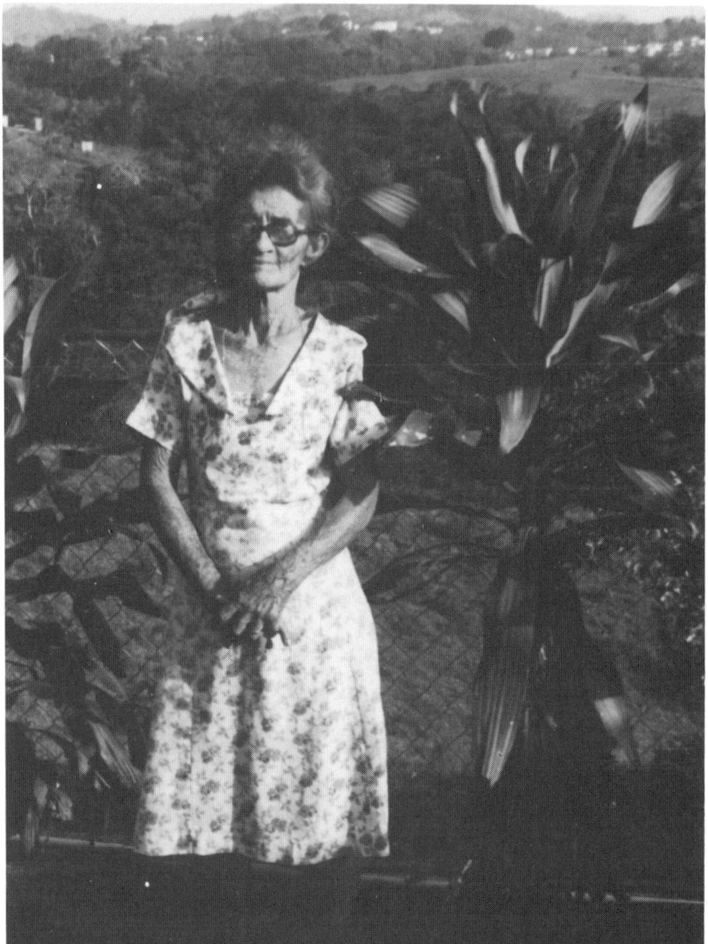

Cruz María Santiago

A Humble Medicine of Earth and Spirit

Cruz María Santiago of Morovis

Doña Cruz María is 73 years old and lives with her husband don Aurelio Santiago González in the outskirts of Morovis. She has brought up twelve children, and has experienced the joy of seeing them all married. At last count, there were nearly a dozen cows, 50 chickens and many medicinal plants sharing the Santiago farm.

Cruz María has the gift of making much out of little, and she creates medicinal products out of wild plants and also foods such as lemon, salt and eggs. Always ready to help her neighbors, here she offers readers a glimpse of her humble yet effective medicines, born of earth and spirit, faith, and plenty of good humor.

Cruz María: I was born here, I grew up here, and I'll die here. The only way I'll leave this place is if they drag me, feet first. Because I'm never leaving Morovis.

M: With twelve children and 73 years of experience, I'll bet you know lots of home remedies. Can you tell me about them?

Cruz María: I used to send the kids out to look for stinging vine (*pringamosa*), which makes an excellent remedy for erysipelas, a terrible inflammation of the skin that burns like crazy.

You have to pick the vine leaves with gloves, because they sting, then you cook some up in oil over a very low flame for five or ten minutes, until the oil turns green. Then you use a feather to paint the oil all over the inflamed area. And that little plant really works! I've used stinging vine to cure three of my kids when they had erysipelas. And I never had to take my kids to the doctor, even with the terrible fever that comes with that condition.

One time, my whole urinary tract felt sore. My kidneys were inflamed, and there was even blood in my urine! Well, I just happened to have three *prenetaria* plants growing outside of my kitchen, and I used them and a piece of spineless (*tuna*) cactus to make a tea. That cured me. I took it whenever I was thirsty, as if it were just plain water, and I can tell you that I've never had another urinary problem. That *prenetaria* is really medicine. I made a tea out of it that time, but you can also prepare it raw. You just wash it and add it to a jar of water and let it sit in your refrigerator. And you can drink as much of that tisane as you like.

M: It can't do any harm . . .

Cruz María: Harm? Never! There used to be a physician around here named Dr. Izquierdo. And whenever anyone had a kidney complaint, he prescribed *prenetaria*.

And that plant has always grown around here. One day, I was opening the gate over there in that corner, and I notice that the *prenetaria* is really looking sparse. I say to God, "Look, with your help, I'm going to pull it out and transplant it in the broadleaf coriander (*recao*) garden." So that's what I did. And the plants have multiplied so now I have a little mountain of them growing, all I could ever need.

M: On the way in, I noticed a good sized *salvia* bush.

Cruz María: My mother always had a bandage of hot *salvia* leaves stuck to her forehead and temples with ointment because she roasted coffee beans, and it was very bad for her. It gave her terrible headaches, and the *salvia* helped her.

M: A few days ago I stayed with a family in Las Marías, and the lady of the house, who also roasts coffee, suffers from terrible headaches as well.

Cruz María: Roasting coffee is simply dangerous! But *salvia* leaves, wrapped around the head like a bandage, make a good remedy for those headaches. And drinking *salvia* as a tea is very good for the throat, especially when you're hoarse. Or you can chew the leaf buds. *Salvia* is a good heating plant when one has a cold.

M: Did you plant this *salvia* bush?

Cruz María: Around here, no one plants it. The birds have brought me the seeds, and here it grows.

M: Some mutual friends have told me that you have an excellent remedy for ringworm.

Cruz María: I treat it with dumb cane (*rábano cimarrón*), the kind that doesn't have any white spots on the leaves. But you have to be careful because just a drop of that juice in your eyes will burn and can even blind you! You cut the burning quality by adding salt to the cane. Incredible, isn't it? Just cut a six or eight-inch piece of dumb cane the long way and put some salt into the cut. If you have large grains of salt, three of four grains will do, but you have to smash them up first. Then you leave it all outside overnight so that it will absorb the cool, damp night air. During that time, the salt dissolves into the liquid from the cane, and in the morning you paint the ringworm with that liquid using a feather. It burns a little but that's how ringworm is cured. No, I never took my kids to a doctor, not for any reason!

You know, at times I even cure myself with lemon. I use lemon for gargles. Because when there's an inflammation of the throat, the lemon's coolness helps a lot. Lemon is medicine.

Look, just last Monday I got out of bed and I couldn't swallow my own saliva. It was as if I had a ball in my throat. And I, imagining the worst, say to myself, "Could this be cancer? It must be a punishment. . . ." But then I realized, "Wait a minute, it can't be a punishment because I haven't done anything wrong!"

So I went to the kitchen and I squeezed some lemon juice into a cup with a little water and added some white vinegar and salt. Then every once in a while I took the cup and gargled. I kept at it all through the night. The hot water cleansed and soothed my throat, and that problem didn't even last two days. It just disappeared, thank God.

And when the cows' teeth get loose, lemon juice tightens them right up. You squeeze everything out of a lemon and add some salt and sugar. Then you rub it along their gums, and don't give them water right away. Now if you don't have lemons around, you can use iodine. That's how I treat the cows. You see, they're chewing greens all the time, so they've always got to be pushing those jaws to work.

Just a little while ago, one of the cows had some loose teeth and she was getting skinny, fast. So I said to Quito, "Leave me alone with her, I'm going to give her some lemon." But the lemon tree had already been harvested. So I went for the iodine, which I always have around. I passed that iodine liquid along her gums with a feather and I left it a while because cows like the flavor. And that tightens their teeth right up. My uncle used to prepare lemons for the cows by roasting them. After they exploded from the heat, he'd let them cool and then pass them, mixed with salt and sugar, all along the gums.

M: I guess just about everyone has lemons at home or can buy them pretty cheaply.

Cruz María: Lemons and salt too. There are times that I cut myself or something else will happen to me, and you'll see me with a little bit of salt water. I just wash myself with salt water, nothing more, and look: all these bumps I have here from dealing with the chickens. I'm all marked up! And that's how I treat myself: water with salt.

Salt water even cured my grandson when that old dog—who is now hidden below—bit him. You see, I have a bunch of cows over there, and we have a watering trough made of cement. Paco was fixing the trough because every morning after they're milked, the cows have to be able to drink their fill of water. Well my grandson is never still and he was running back and forth from the trough to the house here. During one of those trips, I think he must have hit the dog or maybe he tried to put his hand where he shouldn't have. Girl, that dog jumped on top of him, and when I heard that boy yelling and that dog like a fury . . . I was washing dishes. I threw down my dish towel fast, you can believe, and when I got to where they were, the dog was still on top of him. I separated them, brought the boy up to the bathroom, and there I gave him a salt water bath.

That was Monday or Tuesday, and on Friday he was already better. Paco took him to the doctor and the doctor said, "God, you healed quickly!"

You know, that dog has bitten six people, but everyone he bites comes to me, so I can wash them with salt water. And they're all just fine! (laughter)

M: What proportions of water and salt do you use?

Cruz María: Salt water for a bath or to drink means the saltiness of half a cup of water with a teaspoon or so of salt. I always taste the water to make sure it's salty enough because it's the salt that's so medicinal.

They even use salt water when they castrate the pigs! After the operation, they wash'em with salt water so that they don't get tetanus. Salt water is the best thing for almost any condition.

For the teeth! Look, the other day I went to the dentist so that he could pull a tooth. The next day I couldn't even touch my mouth. That whole side was all swollen up. I couldn't eat. My mouth began to twist to one side. And how I suffered at night! The next day I said to myself, "If I were someone else, I'd go and form a labyrinth," because nowadays people will sue for any little thing. But I'm not that kind of person. Then I said, "Wait just a minute!" And I took a little salt and some water and I boiled it right up. I took a mouthful and kept it in my mouth for a good long while. And the next day, when I pressed the gum, a stream of pus came out plus part of my molar that the dentist had left behind. So, thanks to God and the salt water, I got rid of that piece of tooth, the swelling went down, I went to bed, had a good night's sleep and the pain was gone! Just plain water with salt. Salt water is the best thing in the world.

M: Can you talk more about some of the medicinal plants you use?

Cruz María: The broadleaf coriander I cultivate here is just for cooking, but some people use mouthfuls of the boiled root tea to help loosen a tooth for pulling.

And there's all sorts of black nightshade (*mata gallina*) growing around here, although I never planted it. Sometimes people come to look for it here because when you have no control over your stomach—you know, when you've got a diarrhea caused by heat—there's nothing better than black nightshade with *sal de heno* (a sodium bicarbonate-based digestive). If you eat something at night that affects you the next day, boil up the black nightshade for tea, add the *sal de heno* and drink it first thing in the morning on an empty stomach. Black nightshade is the best there is.

Once I got sick on a Monday. I didn't sleep that day nor that night, nor the next day or night. In fact it was Thursday when my husband, who was off to San Juan, said, "I'll leave the city early Friday afternoon so I can take you to the doctor." That's when I remembered the black nightshade, which doesn't cost a penny. I simmered some up until the water was dark green. Then I added the *sal de heno* and I drank it, very strong. And that remedy cured me so well that now I don't even know what it is to have a stomach ache.

At times black nightshade disappears from where it's been growing, but right now, with all the rain that's fallen, you see it right alongside of you everywhere you walk. You prepare a planter with flowers or other plants, and black nightshade springs up right beside them.

Of course, the ideal thing is to have some *tautúa* growing around too, because black nightshade mixed with *tautúa* makes an even better medicine. You can also add it to enemas for children or they can take it as tea. It's cooling and it settles the stomach when you're feeling a little "off."

And right over there, I used to have a tomato plant, which is also medicinal.

M: You use the tomatoes themselves?

Cruz María: No. You heat the leaves and place them with some beef tallow (*sebo de Flandes*) and egg yolk on boils and growths so that they'll explode.

And that same tallow is very good when you have swollen glands. You massage them with the tallow and they go down. One thing's for sure, if it doesn't cure you, you know it certainly hasn't done you any damage. People used to use tallow for mumps too, and for inflamed corns. Even for inflamed pimples on the face. They rubbed that tallow back and forth and the pimples disappeared, little by little.

Another little story just occured to me. My daughter Adelita, the one who lives in New York City, had a boil under her arm that was this big (joins her thumb and index finger to form an OK sign). Since it was located in her armpit, she had to sleep with her arm above her head. My God, was that cyst ugly, and I didn't have the means to take her to the doctor. Suddenly it came to me: an egg! I put the white aside, and using a piece of tissue paper, I painted that red boil with egg yolk. Beneath her, I put a bunch of towels in case it exploded. And it did explode the next day. So I didn't have to bring her to the doctor that time either. Cured by the yolk of an egg!

M: Who taught you that remedy?

Cruz María: It was like a whim that just came to me. I guess the shape of the cyst itself suggested an egg.

M: Have you used egg yolk for any other conditions?

Cruz María: It's also good to make a punch with when someone has a bad chest cold. You beat a fresh egg white and separately you beat the yolk and then they get heated, but you have to keep beating them so that they don't cook. You add almond oil, cinammon, sweet ginger, cloves, anise, everything you have around the house. Because those warming spices are good for a cold and flu.

I don't know. It seems to me that nowadays people get worse colds and flu than before. People today seem to get sicker more often too, although we weren't so hygiene conscious then as we are now. You see that I had a big family and they grew up healthy and strong. I never took those kids to a doctor. If they had a cough, I gave them a rub with some warm Vicks and I made them some spiced eucalyptus (*eucalipto*) or ginger (*jengibre dulce*) tea. And they never got asthma or anything!

Well, that's about all I know, I guess. Anyway, I've got to get off to church now.

M: Seems to me you know a great deal. Thanks so much!

Cruz María: May God and the Virgin Mary bless you.

Beauticians and Neighbors of Carolina

Ana Clausells de Costoso, Josefina Pizarro,
María Salgado,
Julia Santiago, Monín Santana

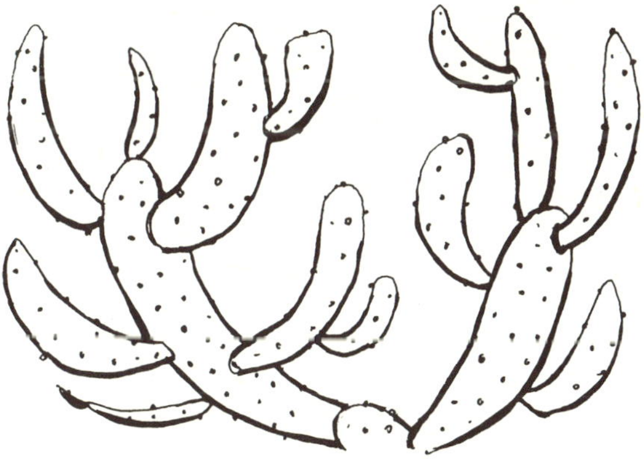

spineless tuna cactus *la tuna*

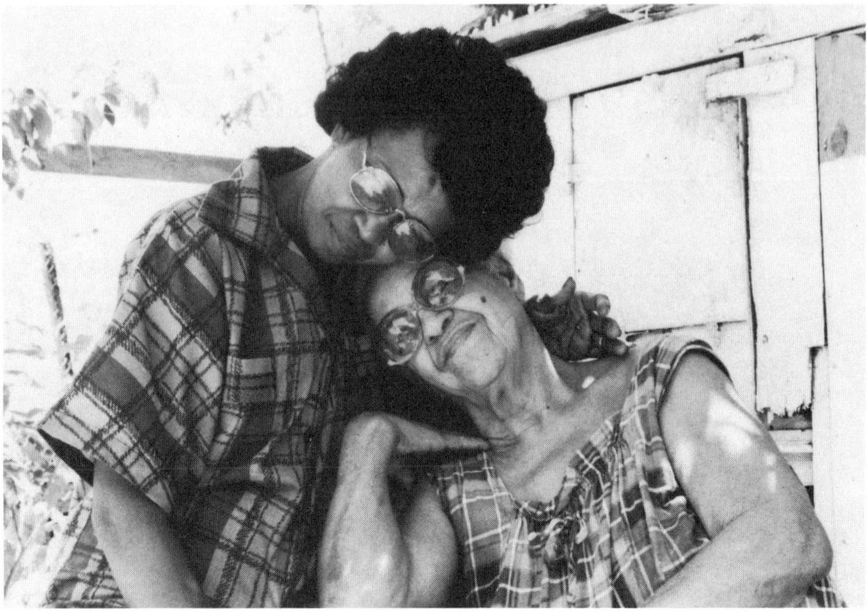

Ana Clausells de Costoso and Julia Santiago

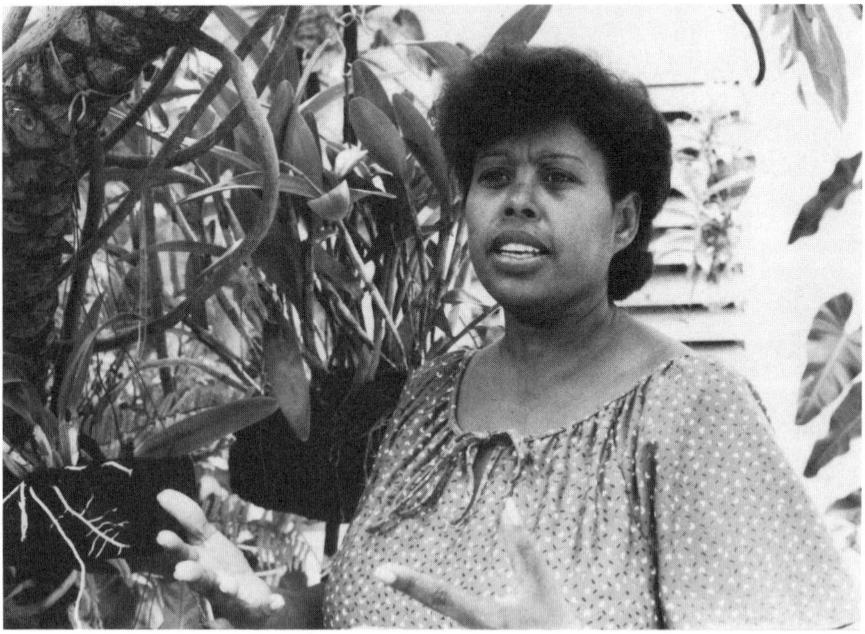

Josefina Pizarro

Beauticians and Neighbors of Carolina

Ana Clausells de Costoso, Josefina Pizarro, María Salgado, Julia Santiago, Monín Santana

Ana Clausells de Costoso and Josefina Pizarro are housewives and mothers who also share the responsibilities of a beauty parlor at Ana's home, part of a peaceful community in Carolina. They speak from experience about plant-based beauty products as well as medicine.

Our interview flowed with the informality of a neighborly visit as one of their clients, María Salgado, and two very dear neighbors, Julia Santiago and Monín Santana, generously contributed their knowledge. The conversation took place at both Ana's and Julia's homes, and our talk was punctuated by delicious sips of Ana's homemade tamarind ices and the lively sound of doña Julia's roosters.

M: Doña Ana, your son Carlos Alberto told me that you use plants as medicine, cosmetics, and even to get rid of ticks!

Ana: Yes, we use *poleo* for that. If there are ticks around, you put all the poleo that fits—leaves without stems—into a bucket of water. The stronger the better, but you don't boil it.

You simply leave the *poleo* there to steep from one day to the next, and then you pour it in and around the doghouse or wherever the ticks are. The water has a strong smell, and the ticks will move on quickly.

María: *Poleo* is also good for a stomach ache. When something I've eaten disagrees with me, I go down to the garden and pick some *poleo* and *guanábana* leaves for tea. The discomfort goes away immediately after drinking it.

Ana: There were eight kids in my family, and when we had stomach aches, my mother used to give us a tea of budding mango leaves mixed with *guanábana* leaves. And it always worked. You see, since they're both cooling, they reduce the acid in your stomach.

Josefina: Not too long ago, everyone knew about medicinal plants, but along with progress, a lot of information was forgotten. Suddenly now, with the come-back of naturism, the plants are being rediscovered. For example, everyone knows that aloe vera (*sábila*) is good for a cough. You peel some thick aloe leaves, cut the inside gelatin up in pieces, put it in a bowl with a little witch hazel solution and some honey, and let it sit for a day or so, so that the plant's medicinal qualities are dissolved in the liquid. You take tablespoons of it, all mixed up like that, and it loosens the phlegm from your chest.

Ana: One of my mother's favorite remedies for a cough was the papaya flower. I still boil it up myself and add honey. It's very effective.

María: *Malá* is also good for getting rid of phlegm from your lungs, especially for people who have asthma. You boil up two of the succulent leaves with a few anise stars in a cup and a half of water for about fifteen minutes, and then you drink it. That gets rid of phlegm and blood too.

You know, I was born ill, and as an infant I was in a great deal of pain. My father thought I wouldn't last even a few weeks! He had me baptized right away so that I wouldn't die a "heathen," as they say; but my mother cured me with plants, and I never went to a doctor when I was a child.

You know what they gave me when I had the measles? Love vine (*afilerillo*). It has a little white flower and it grows up to fifty feet high. My mother prepared cooling drinks of love vine, which took away the burning heat that coursed through me. Thanks to *mamá*, I was cured of the measles within one week.

Josefina: When I had the measles, my mother gave me boiled milk with raisins. For that kind of inner heat condition, it was a wonderfully cooling remedy. It drew the measles right out of me, fast.

Other times, my mom put raw rice in water and left it there for an hour or more. Now it's coming back to me. She gave us rice water for stomach ache and for diarrhea. It was a different kind of rice in those days; the grains were very long.

M: The hulls of brown rice and other whole grains are loaded with water-soluble B vitamins, which tonify both the intestinal tract and the nervous system.

Josefina: It's amazing how much our mothers knew, just through their experience!

Ana: My mother used rice water for her skin. She would let raw rice sit in a little bit of water, then grind it up to make a paste. In fact, we all made facial masks from that paste, and it kept our complexions really clean. I *never* got pimples.

M: Can you talk more about using plants as cosmetics?

Ana: I've used Caribbean vervain (*verbena*) on my daughter's hair to help it grow. I boil it, let it cool off, wash her hair, and then I pour the vervain "tea" over her hair and leave it there. You can add any conditioner you like but you must leave the vervain there. She had hardly any hair growing out of the back of her head, and now she has a mane!

Actually I've recommended that three of my clients with the same problem go out to the plaza and buy some vervain. After using it a while, they've all had good results.

M: I've heard about using Caribbean vervain as a fever remedy, but I never heard anyone talk about it as a cure for scant hair. I'm sure lots of people will be trying it out!

Josefina: We also use rosemary (*romero*) boiled up as a final rinse. It adds body and gives your hair a nice dark color.

Ana: I use aloe vera gel to give hair body too, and it's great for getting rid of dandruff. I just peel a large stalk, cut it up into tiny pieces, put them in three or four cups of water and leave it all in the refrigerator. The next day, I beat the mixture, strain it, and apply it to the hair after shampooing. I never rinse it out. You don't have to boil it, and if you make a decent quantity of it, it can stay in the refrigerator for future rinses; it doesn't go bad right away.

M: Aloe vera is an amazing plant.

María: So is the spineless (*tuna*) cactus. Believe it or not, they charge $3 for just one leaf of it in New York! You simply peel it, cut it up, and put it in water in a jar in the refrigerator. Then, instead of drinking water from the faucet, you drink the cactus water. It's a tisane that cools the kidneys and increases urination.

M: By tisane, you mean an herbal preparation that hasn't been boiled?

Ana: Yes. When we say tisane we mean a raw plant in water, "brewed" in the fridge. The juice of the plant dissolves little by little into the water. Some people also put their boiled teas in the refrigerator to drink cold, but that's different. A tisane is made without heat.

María: I also prepare tisanes from a little plant called *prenetaria*. It grows wild all over the place, wherever there's humidity, even through the cracks in the sidewalk! I just pick it, wash it, put it in a jar of water in the fridge, and drink it to clean out my kidneys.

There are medicinal plants for everything, even the heart! The leaves of the custard apple tree (*corazón*) can be boiled up for a tea that's said to strengthen the heart as it lowers blood pressure.

I don't know. It seems that living in the city, you really tend to forget these good old remedies of the past!

Ana: But even scientists are still using plants as a source of medicine.

M: Scientists use the part or parts of a plant which they've determined to be most useful, but I believe that all parts of a plant are useful. They have so much to offer: minerals, vitamins, fiber, and a number of compounds which work together in a natural and perfect way . . .

Ana: They may be perfect, but some plants not only cure; they can also kill.

María: I know a plant that can kill. It has an exquisite flower, but you can die from drinking a tea of it. It's called the moon plant (*campana*).

Ana: Another plant that both heals and kills is black nightshade (*mata gallina*). The seed is poison, but the leaf boiled in milk cures ulcers!

Josefina: Actually, the seed is a purgative. Which reminds me of castor oil, another great purgative that was also used for intestinal worms. Nowadays it doesn't have much of a smell, but back then it was real "natural," if you know what I mean! (laughter)

And the leaves of the castor bean plant (*higuereta*) were boiled up to make sitz baths for women suffering from congestion or inflammation of the womb area. After boiling a big handful of leaves in a large pot for 15 minutes, you strain the liquid and pour it into the warm bath water. Then you sit there for ten or fifteen minutes or until you feel better.

Ana: After giving birth, we women used to drink a mixture of real, bittersweet chocolate boiled with red mint (*yerba buena*). You simply boil half a bar of that chocolate with two cups of water and add eight or ten leaves of red mint to help strengthen the womb after birth.

M: I'll bet lots of women enjoyed drinking that medicine.

Josefina: Right! Not all home remedies are like castor oil! (laughter)

M: Besides castor oil and other strong purgatives, what are some other remedies for constipation?

Josefina: A tea made from the young leaves of *tártago*. But you have to make the tea out of new leaf buds because the mature parts of the plant contain poisons. It's one of the plants that can both cure and kill. The seed is poison, but the young bud cures constipation. I've given it to my daughter Maura and it really works.

Doña María had come for a beauty parlor appointment, and now her husband has arrived to pick her up, calling with long, steady beeps of his car horn. After she leaves, amidst many goodbyes and blessings, Ana and Josefina take me back into the patio garden, where broadleaf coriander, prenetaria, life plant, native lentils and aloe vera grow alongside trees bearing abundant oranges, lemons, guanábanas and custard apples.

Ana: Do you know about the life plant (*bruja*)? It's the best thing in the world for an earache. You warm up the leaf on the heat of the stove, and squeeze out the warm juice into your ear. You can cover it up with some cotton afterwards, but it's not always necessary. And life plant is special for another reason. If you hang one of the leaves up from a tack on a wall, it will sprout roots without ever touching the earth!

Oh, and the native lentil (*gandul*) leaf can be used when there's no toothpaste. It cleans the teeth and strengthens the gums. You just place the leaf against the gums and rub as if it were a little brush.

M: I love hearing about plants that offer both medicine and food.

Ana: Well then you should know that the spineless (*tuna*) cactus we mentioned earlier makes a delicious stewed vegetable. It's something like okra. First you peel it, than you cook it up with garlic, onion, vegetables and cod fish or meat. I had some for the first time over at doña Julia's house and I didn't even realize it was tuna cactus. It's delicious, and it's got a nice, fat little texture!

Speaking of food, lemon in warm salt water makes a great gargle. Because the salt cleanses the throat, and the lemon has vitamin C.

strain it and add it to your bath. It cools, cleans, and alleviates inflammation too.

Another remedy for the same condition is a bath of wild eggplant leaves (*berenjena cimarrona*). You prepare it the same way as the plantain bath and then you just sit for a while in that water, while it's fairly warm. It helps a lot.

Ana: Doña Julia, what's that herb you use for wounds and sores?

Julia: *Yerba cangá*, dried. After you've washed the wound well, you sprinkle the pulverized leaf dust on it.

Ana: And when children get constipated?

Julia: When my kids had that problem, I always started out by giving them a teaspoon of cooking oil. Then I rubbed the hairs off a few stems of *cohitre blanco*, pressed the stems into a little ball, and covered it with oil before using it as a suppository. That's a good children's remedy.

Monín: For constipation you can also mix the sap of a leaf of aloe vera with a washed and chopped leaf of spineless tuna cactus in the blender with two cups of water. Add honey and drink it throughout the day. Plus, eat fresh, natural food with lots of fiber. Nothing canned.

If a child gets indigestion, you can give him a remedy of wood ashes. My mother used to take wood ashes from the cooking stove and put a pinch of those ashes in a cup of water. She let them settle for a while, and then the child would drink that water with half a teaspoonful of cooking oil.

M: Now they sell charcoal capsules at the store for gas and indigestion. It comes in a modern capsule, but it's probably one of our most ancient medicines.

Monín: Charcoal is also good for absorbing odors in the refrigerator. So many of the old country ways are still valuable.

M: What did you all do when your children got high fevers?

Monín: We gave them special baths with plants.

Julia: For an unboiled bath, we would squeeze the juice of fresh aloe, *poleo*, mugwort (*altamisa*), garlic weed (*anamú*) and everything else we could find into a bucket of water. Then we added some alcohol to the water and put it outside in a strong sun. Within half an hour it was ready for a bath. We have a camphor tree here, but if there are no camphor (*alcanfor*) leaves around, you can add half a camphor pastille to the water and that makes it even fresher. After straining the bath, we poured it over the child's head. Then the child would get all wrapped up so that he could sweat as much as possible.

M: Are there food products which you use as remedies?

Julia: If you use a poultice of grated potato directly after burning yourself, you'll see that the burn doesn't get a blister, and you might not even lose any hair from the burned spot!

Potato is also good for really bad headaches. Just grate it and mix it up with some witch hazel solution *(Agua Maravilla)* to make a cooling paste. Put it on your forehead and temples and neck, and lie down for a little while. What a delicious feeling! Pure relief! You're revived. And I'm speaking from experience.

Ana: You have a remedy for diabetes, don't you?

Julia: Yes, mulberry leaves (*morera*). Boil up five leaves for fifteen minutes in about three cups of water, and drink it every day. I have diabetes and it's really helped me. And when I used to work as a nurse, I had a diabetic patient who was really sick. I told her, "Don't worry. Tomorrow I'm going to bring you a little mulberry tea, and that will take care of your condition." So I came home and boiled up some mulberry leaves and took her a big jar of it the next day. She hid the jar in her suitcase and every once in a while she took a swig. Well, when they checked her blood sugar, they found that it was quite low. Believe me, when she went home, the doctor told her to keep taking that "secret remedy" she'd been hiding, because it was extremely effective.

Monín: Doctors are aware. They realize that people have their own resources.

M: If someone is always tired, sleepy, and very low on energy, what would you recommend?

Julia: I'd suggest that she take a hemoglobin or red blood count. If it comes out low, I would suggest that she make lots of punches from all the most nourishing and strengthening things: grape juice, orange juice, malt. If the problem is a simple matter of fatigue from doing too much physical work, I would recommend a heavier diet and I'd suggest drinking lots of broth. Of course the best thing is always dove or pigeon broth. After drinking that, almost immediately you feel a tremendous surge of energy, and you say, "Yes I can!" Keep drinking it for two or three weeks, and you get "strong as a palm tree," as they say in the country. Strong and resistant.

M: Those roosters are really something. How do you treat them when they get sick?

Julia: When they or the chickens get "the pip," which is contagious and leaves then with that heavy mucous, I just add lemon juice to their water. That takes care of it.

Ana: Look at her life plants!

M: They are really big and beautiful.

Julia: You know, when you pass by a plant you really must greet it. You have to say, "Good morning beautiful." If it's a life plant, maybe you say, "Give me a little leaf to help me out with this ear that's hurting." You should talk to it as if it were a person, as if it had a soul. Because if you have a plant and you tend it every day, giving it water, watching it grow, and wishing it well, that plant will become your friend.

M: Your *salvia* plant looks pretty happy!

Julia: I've always made teas out of *salvia*. It's very good for menstrual pains. Because those pains come from a cold condition, and *salvia* is warming.

Ana: Tell her about the butter poultice . . .

Julia: When you've bruised yourself and the bruise starts swelling, use a poultice of butter, salt and sugar to bring the swelling right down. You just mix equal amounts of butter and sugar with about half the amount of salt. Put it all on top of the wound, and there will be no swelling.

M: I love to hear about remedies like this, because even if someone doesn't have a garden, everyone has a little butter, salt and sugar in the house.

Julia: That's true . . . and there's also faith, which doesn't cost a thing.

You know, before they operated on my eyes, everything I saw was in a blur. I couldn't thread a needle, so I couldn't do any mending. I couldn't even tend to the plants because, practically speaking, I was blind. But one of my neighbors held a service at her house. Alicia and Ana here prayed for me, and I felt a marked difference afterwards. I can't say I could see perfectly the next day, but I came back here and worked with the plants and took care of my clothes. What could be greater or more beautiful than that?

M: You have a lot of faith in home-made medicines too, don't you?

Julia: Yes, I take my medicinal teas and other home remedies. I drink everything folks offer me, and I do it with the faith that it will help me. Some people say, "I'll try this remedy and see if it does anything for me." But I say, "They're giving me this medicinal tea and it's second only to God." I've always believed in home remedies, and I've come to trust them more and more because they've really worked for me!

Planting with the Moon in Caguas

Panky Negrón Maldonado

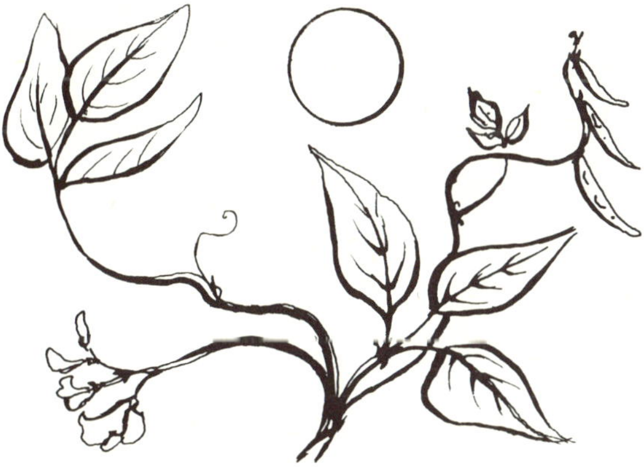

native bean *habichuelas del país*

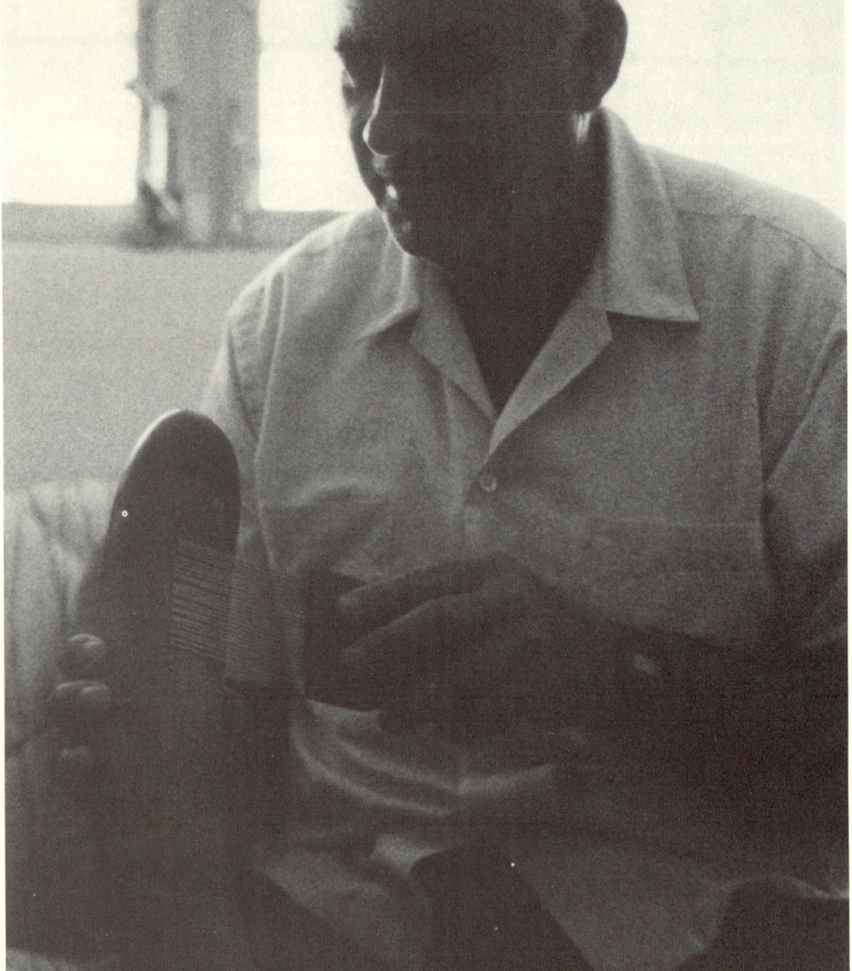

"Panky" Negrón Maldonado

Planting with the Moon in Caguas

Panky Negrón Maldonado

Not so very long ago, when the Puerto Rican people lived on food produced by their own labor on island soil, Panky Negrón Maldonado learned about working the land in the fields of Vega Alta. Trailing after his father and a pair of oxen, he learned to prepare the soil, to plant each seed and seedling at the proper depth, and to sow and harvest different vegetables at the most propitious times. According to his father, there is a time of year and even a time of month for planting almost everything that grows in Puerto Rico. Leonardo Negrón Santiago worked in harmony with the moon and the tides; he taught his son to do the same.

Since he left the farm when he was 17, Panky has made a living in urban settings, mostly as a police officer. But he has always maintained a small piece of land, where he grows several vegetables for his table, and abundant crops of tender native beans (*habichuelas del país*).

The once-ubiquitous, cream-colored native bean is almost impossible to find today because of a recent shift in agricultural and consumer practices. Thus, they are the envy of his neighbors and the delight of co-workers and friends who buy the surplus.

Panky is a sophisticated, well-traveled individual, but his love for the earth and his understanding about planting are part of an island-based tradition of building and tending healthy, fertile soil in balance with nature.

Panky: The most valuable thing my father taught me in terms of agriculture is that nothing should be planted when the moon is new or waxing. If you break this basic rule, your plants will be tender just when the insects are hungriest, so you'll lose a great portion of your crops. The solution is to plant during the waning moon. That way, when the insects are ready to eat, the plants are no longer vulnerable. I've always planted during the waning moon, and I've had tremendous results.

I sow native beans on a tiny piece of land about 300 metres square, and from that piece of land I easily harvest 70 or 80 pounds of beans every time I plant. The last time I planted was in February, and I had my best crop, harvesting more than 80 pounds in April. I was able to give away and sell 40 pounds of the beans! Then from the money I earned by selling them, I bought fertilizer. The other half of my crop is packed away in the freezer. They'll last me until the next crop is ready, in July.

M: What kind of fertilizer do you use?

Panky: I use natural fertilizers. There's a company here in Puerto Rico that packages the rich alluvial soil which is deposited along the river beds. That alluvium is then mixed with other soils, and it's great for the plants. Manure is also very good fertilizer. Chicken manure is one of the richest, but its nitrogen content is so high that if it's used before it sits for a year or two, it actually burns the plants. And what a smell! I brought some home once, and Margarita almost kicked me out (laughter). So it's got to be "cured."

M: Do you follow the same rule of planting with the moon for everything you plant, or are there exceptions?

Panky: Actually, yucca and sugar cane can be planted at any time of month. They're both virtually immune to insect infestation, no matter when they're planted. But they're the only plants that have this quality, as far as I know.

On the other hand, when planting plantains and bananas, you want to observe not only the phases of the moon; you also want to work with the tide. Each tree produces six or seven seeds, which must be taken during low tide; otherwise the seed is all wet and loses its sap. You want to take the seed when it's driest; that way it maintains its essence, and has the capacity to absorb the most from the earth.

Old-time farmers used to be able to tell whether it was high or low tide simply by looking at the veins on their hands. If the veins were swollen, it was high tide; if they were flat, it was low tide. I never used my hands in that way, but from my own experience, I can tell you that it's very important to collect the plantain and banana seeds when the tide is low if you want an optimum yield from your trees. And then, of course, you plant the seeds during the waning moon.

M: Have you actually experimented with planting seeds at different times of month and taking banana tree seeds, let's say, during high tide?

Panky: Of course. Everything I'm telling you I've proven for myself. Nothing comes from books or lectures. I've experimented with taking seeds at high tide and I've tried planting seeds during the waxing moon. Basically, I've seen that plants seeded when the moon is waxing may sprout beautifully, but they won't yield a thing, because when they're about to produce their fruit, they're eaten by the insects. It's a disaster.

M: What insects are these?

Panky: There are several. The worst threat is *la esperanza* (a type of grasshopper) at the larval stage, but there are several moths and flying insects which lay their eggs on the plants or in the earth near them. The eggs hatch, and you never see them while they're in their larval stage because they burrow into the earth. They do a great deal of damage unless you plant at the proper time.

People think that these old ways of farming are unnecessary. They say, "On the big farms in the United States, they don't plant by the moon." But they forget that on those big farms, airplanes spray insecticide all over the crops.

M: The bad thing is that the insecticide contaminates the earth and poisons the people.

Panky: And we don't know the effects of these poisons for the future. Plus, in many cases, insects actually develop immunity to the chemicals designed to kill them. Who knows? Maybe eventually, there won't be anything that kills them . . . without killing us first (laughter).

M: Do you ever use insecticide?

Panky: I have used it, but I've gotten the best results when I haven't. This year, for instance, I didn't use anything, and I didn't see any insects; nothing! So I saved money, and the soil is better off.

Living on the Land

Cheo y Bárbara Rodríguez

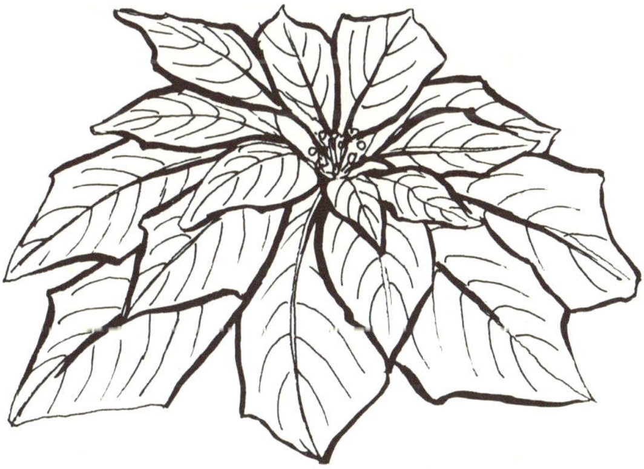

poinsettia *la pascua*

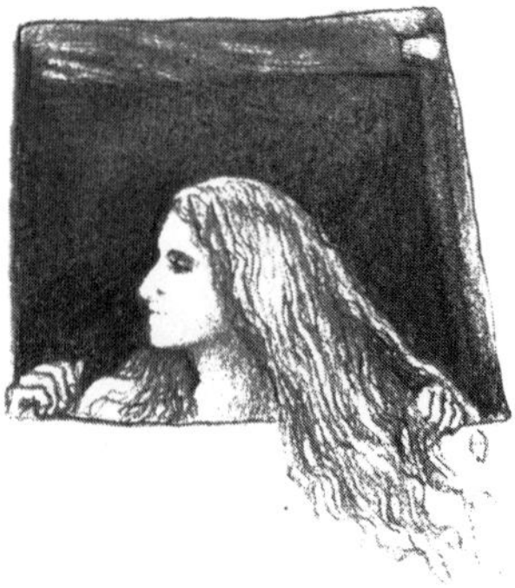

In the mountains

Living on the Land

Cheo y Bárbara Rodríguez

Cheo and Bárbara Rodríguez live in the mountainous, central part of the island, tucked away about an hour's hike from the nearest paved road, with no phone and no TV. Since 1973, they have lived as close to the land as possible, working the soil in return for food and a vast array of medicinal plants. They avoid most animal products and stay as close to traditional foods as possible, which means lots of *viandas* (root vegetables such as celery root, yucca, yautía and malanga), plenty of regional vegetables, fruits, whole grains, seeds, and pure, flowing stream water which has been routed to flow right through their kitchen. They are deeply concerned with the cultural integrity of Puerto Rico, and share thoughts about how this integrity is related to and reflected in the diet, health, attitudes, and agriculture of her people. They are committed to learning about, cultivating and using medicinal plants, practices which were once part of Puerto Rico's daily cultural expression.

M: Living here in the country, so far away from the mainstream of society, what has been your motivation or inspiration, and what are your goals?

Cheo: When we moved here, my goal was to strengthen my own health and to test my belief that my physical problems were greatly due to the environment in which I lived. And coming to a healthy environment *has* helped me to become healthy again.

Bárbara: All of my family comes from the mountains, so when I was a child, I got lots of exposure to country life and life in small towns. Then my parents moved to the city, where I remained till I was 18. But when I came back to the country as an adult, I felt at home once more. It was a matter of falling in love with something that I'd already known. That's been my inspiration. My goal now is to raise my family in a healthy environment.

M: Can you talk about your relationship with the earth and with the plants, especially?

Cheo: We keep in mind the fact that each one of us is part of everything, and we're involved in discovering relationships between ourselves and everything else. Even though we're distant from our human neighbors, we're surrounded by all the living creatures in the mountains, including the plants. And they offer us friendship, food, joy, health, life!

Bárbara: Without green plants in our lives, we couldn't survive; we'd die and become earth ourselves, so they're all important. Plants are very special beings. They live in a dimension parallel to our own, and they are here to help us.

Cheo: People used to live in such close quarters with nature, with the plants. And you can see that closeness in the beauty and strength of our grandparents and great grandparents. We're trying to rediscover that which worked so well in the past.

Bárbara: One thing we've discovered is that the plants used for health, be they food or medicine, aren't exotic or strange. They grow wild right outside your front door; they're from the environment you live in, sharing energy with you. When we live in cities, we forget that we're sharing the world with them.

My great grandmother always had all kinds of medicinal plants growing in her garden. She never ran to the doctor for pills or injections. In those days, everyone used the medicinal plants growing in their gardens; they knew how to prepare them because their parents and grandparents and their great grandparents had done it. The knowledge passed from one person to another, from one generation to another.

Every *jíbaro* household had its garden, and every garden had its red mint (*yerba buena*), marjoram (*mejorana*), rosemary (*romero*), peppermint (*menta*), lemon grass (*limoncillo*), rue (*ruda*), fragrant geranium (*geranio oloroso*), *paletaria*. They were an important part of the household. In what looked like an ornamental flower garden, you could find medicine for just about everything. If you felt ill, you didn't go anywhere; someone prepared you a little *guarapo* or they fixed you a hot bath and wrapped you up in warm blankets so that you could sweat. Women generally guarded the information about medicinal plants, while the men were more involved with plants used for food.

But all of that knowledge, which for so long had been passed down from generation to generation, was cut off at the root because another wave of ideas took over completely. The new wave said, "How could you think that a bunch of weeds is really medicine? That's ignorance!" And since no one wants to be ignorant, the old ways were hidden, ignored, forgotten . . . and the new ways became the authority, dominating the entire scene.

We're losing a tremendous amount of this information with the death of our elders, our grandparents, our midwives, the bonesetters, and others. But there are still old people in the countryside and in the villages who will tell you that this plant is good for certain conditions, and that if you mix it with this other plant and make a *guarapo*, you can treat such and such a problem. This information can still be recovered, especially from the oldest people on the island.

M: Do you have favorite plants that you like to work with?

Cheo: The plant that has surprised us the most in terms of its instantaneous effect is comfrey (*consuelda mayor*).

Bárbara: We use it for all kinds of skin irritations. When the youngest was an infant, she was so plump that her little legs were always rubbing against one another; they got pretty badly irritated and soon she had a full-blown rash. I was worried because it simply wouldn't go away no matter what we tried.

Then I got some comfrey, squeezed out some of the slippery juice from the long, thick stems with a rolling pin, and used that juice as an ointment. Well, within ten or fifteen minutes, the irritation disappeared, and the baby was fine! Nothing bothered her at all after that. That was the most dramatic and immediate reaction I've ever seen. Now we use comfrey all the time for skin irritations, and it always soothes.

Then there's garlic (*ajo*)! My grandfather had cancer for about twenty years, it seems, without anyone knowing about it. Instinctively, he ate raw garlic every day. My grandmother hated the smell, so in order not to bother her, he would grind it up, put it in a piece of soft bread, and swallow it like a pill every day. He never missed a day of taking his garlic, and it maintained his strength, his health. When the doctors operated on him, they couldn't figure out how he had lived so long, because the cancer had spread throughout his entire body and even to his brain; meanwhile, he was still completely clear minded and coherent. He could carry on a conversation without your noticing that anything was amiss. The garlic seems to have been responsible for oxygenating his blood and keeping him alive.

M: Garlic is also used by a great number of people for high blood pressure.

Cheo: And raw garlic counteracts the poisonous effects of alcohol.

Bárbara: Garlic doesn't even have to be eaten to be effective. You can wear it, and its antiseptic and other medicinal qualities are absorbed by the skin. And if someone has parasites, a clove of garlic in the rectum will get rid of them fast.

Of course, it smells, whether you eat it or wear it.

Cheo: It was an indigenous custom to hang a clove of garlic around the ankles of small children. It was supposed to keep the poisonous snakes from biting them. They would avoid the smell. Now it's people who avoid the smell. (laughter) Seriously, so many people today are looking for natural ways of balancing out aspects of modern life. Even people who are using drugs can use simple home remedies to make sure that the drugs don't do too much damage. Which reminds me . . . I know someone who, in the process of recovering from cocaine abuse, used lecithin and orange tree leaves (*hojas de naranjo*) to calm himself and strengthen his nervous system; it alleviated what would have been a tremendously difficult period.

Bárbara: Calcium also helps the nerves. You can get it from sesame (*ajonjolí*), from seaweed, from nettle leaves (*ortiga*), from many sources besides milk, and it alleviates anxiety.

Cheo: Of course, lemon (*limón*) is loaded with vitamin C, which can be used to fight the effects even of drugs as strong as heroin. In fact our neighbor, doña Pancha's son, quit alcohol using lemon. Just lemon! So not only did he stop drinking, but the vitamin C strengthened him physically.

Bárbara: It also strengthened his will power, his self esteem, his character. Every time he had the urge to drink alcohol, he drank lemon juice; and since it was as bracing as the alcohol, it allowed him to give up alcohol altogether.

M: I recently heard of an experimental study being done in California in which alcoholics are injected with high dosages of vitamin C. It seems that the vitamin C enables them to stop drinking without withdrawal symptoms.

Cheo: There is a tremendous amount of wisdom in the popular tradition. One day science will catch up! (laughter) I remember once, when I was living in rather primitive conditions, I had an infestation of cockroaches. A beautiful old lady came over and said to me, "Son, cockroaches hate *poleo*. Put branches of it throughout your little home here, and they'll just disappear." I did that, and with only two or three branches in each corner, I got rid of every single cockroach. Just think!

M: An extract of *poleo* would sell like crazy in New York if people knew about it.

Bárbara: (laughter) Plants offer so many possibilities to people: possibilities of maintaining one's health, of healing, of knowing a beautiful part of reality.

M: You know I'm always ready to hear about another home remedy.

Bárbara: There are so many. Did you know that the milky juice of the poinsettia (*pascua*) plant eliminates warts? Just pick a few leaves and apply the milky juice that flows from the cut areas to the warts. They'll disappear after just four or five applications.

Cheo: And the latex-y milk from the green papaya kills intestinal parasites. Cut some long slits into a just-harvested, green papaya. Then, with a teaspoon, collect the white latex that seeps out of the cuts. Since the latex is caustic, you have to mix it with juice so as not to burn your lips. Take a teaspoonful or two a day, always on an empty stomach. Within three days you will have eliminated the parasites. And the same remedy can be used for poor digestion. Just take the latex-like milk mixed with juice after meals.

Bárbara: Nettle is good for many types of fungus that grow on the hands, feet and between the legs. It's even used to cure *la culebrilla* (a painful neuritis that affects the skin). You pick the nettle leaves with a towel so as not to get stung, then you use a mortar and pestle or a rolling pin to crush them. Leave the crushed leaves and juice in water for three or four hours. Later, strain the water and keep it in the refrigerator. Every hour (at least six or seven times a day) wash the ailing area with the nettle water and let it dry in the air, without rubbing. Recuperation time depends on the gravity of the condition, but we've seen some amazing results.

The same nettle water has been used traditionally as a hair rinse to combat dandruff. You simply pour it over the scalp after shampooing, and leave it there without rinsing it off.

Cheo: There are also psychological levels of working with plants, with the symbols involved. For instance, they say that mint (*la menta*) affects *la mente*, the mind.

Bárbara: There are truths buried in so much of our folklore.

M: You use baths and sweats and teas and other herbal preparations to work on the psychological level of healing. Can you talk about how you prepare a bath, for instance?

Cheo: You can prepare a bath with an instruction manual, or you can do it in an improvised way, as if you were a singer inventing verses appropriate to a situation.

There are a great many factors. For instance, we have one plant, *santa María*, which blooms every two, three or five years. Conditions have to be just right or the plant won't flower. So you go out to collect plants for a bath, and you notice, "the *santa María* is in flower; I must take some for my bath," and "over there the *cariaquillo* seems to be beckoning." So you prepare your bath according to what is happening in the moment. It's an intuitive process, but it's based on knowledge.

When you're in charge of helping someone through a bath, you see the thread of ideas and feelings that are welling up in the person. If you know that the person is having love problems, you have some indication of how to go about soothing and easing, and you keep that in your mind when you go out looking for plants for the bath.

Then boil, for 15 or 20 minutes, the leaves, stems, flowers and roots you've chosen, and add them to the person's bath water. Sprinkle some fresh flowers on top. Have the person listen to soothing music while bathing. Help him or her to feel safe and completely taken care of. Then see what happens.

Using plants in therapeutic baths can have long-term effects on many levels.

M: During the three days I've been with you, I've noticed that you're always harvesting fresh vegetables for salad; you even eat salad for breakfast!

Cheo: It's important to eat greens and flowers while they're still vibrating with life. The best way to take in the goodness of the plants is to eat them as fresh as possible, so that their vital essence is maintained. But for our friends who live in the city, we also liquify fresh plants and then freeze the liquid in little ice cubes. It's a good way of preserving their essence and the plants' special properties without having to dry, heat or use alcohol to preserve them. It's an instant lift full of the pure energy of the plants . . . as if you'd just cut and crushed a bunch of fresh plants and put them in your mouth. Delicious, cooling, and nutritious!

M: Can you talk more about the tradition of home-based healing in Puerto Rico?

Bárbara: Besides the presence of backyard medicinal gardens in every home, besides the fact that everyone knew something about using plants for medicine, there was also always someone special in the community who dealt with the most difficult cases. That person would deal on the physical, emotional and spiritual levels all at once. S/he knew and knows that you can't separate a headache from an emotional trouble or frustration, for example. So you went to that person for a blessing, for a rub. You went to that person with the assurance that s/he would help you through her or his energy and good faith.

M: Money was never an object.

Bárbara: No. People would bring eggs or a chicken, some *viandas* or other necessities. But the people involved in healing had no monetary interest. They would give their lives to help people, and they themselves—their dedication, their energy—were part of the medicine. They had a tremendous instinct for healing, and they were totally devoted to their calling. Their motivation was always simply to help, to alleviate pain, to heal.

All this has been made fun of; people laugh and say, "It's witchcraft," or "It's all in the mind; just psychological!" But the psychological aspects of health are very important, and have their place in medicine. The physical has always been related to the psychological and spiritual, to one's intentions, dedication, and thoughts. They've always been one.

M: The relationship between the physical and psychological worlds is being studied seriously today by both scientists and medical professionals on the cutting edge of medical science.

Bárbara: But the typical doctor of today who has invested so much money and spent so many years studying, without even having a life apart from his studies for so many years, wants to live it up a little and feels like a total failure if he gets assigned to a hospital for poor people.

Meanwhile, the people who healed traditionally offered their services for free, from the heart: hot baths, rubs and adjustments, teas. Mostly they were women.

In fact, the healer was also related to the birth giving process in some way. She had to do with everything that was life and health. She was probably a midwife, a *comadrona*. A man in the same role might have been called a *comadrón*. These people were very well respected until the destructive deculturization process started in with its: "You old people don't know anything. Let the professionals from the north teach you about real medicine."

That's how baby formulas found their way to the shelves of new mothers. The people were told it was better than mother's milk. They began to look down on our traditional midwives and healers, who were intimidated by being called "ignorant, uneducated, superstitious, country bumpkins." That brainwashing went on steadily during my grandmother's and my mother's generations. It all happened so fast, and our parents grew up in the new wave. Everyone my mother's age was born at home with a midwife. My mother suckled at my grandmother's breast until she was three years old! During that time, she slept in her parents' bed and went to the neighborhood healers for blessings and therapies, for herbal remedies and spritual healings. These are still tremendous memories for her.

Meanwhile, everyone in my generation was born in the hospital; the bottle was better than the breast; we started out eating commercial baby foods. Modern psychology said that the children should be separated from their parents as soon as possible. Everything was turned upside down in such a short time. It was like a guillotine that cut off people's relationship with tradition at the roots; and it cut off a tremendous amount of knowledge as well.

People would actually deny they knew anything about plants so that they wouldn't be considered ignorant!

Cheo: Medicine is related to everything. We know that when one group of people sets out to destroy another, they prohibit the spiritual practices of the people. And medicine, work with plants, is closely related to those practices.

Destroying popular medicine is a way of weakening a nation. Because popular medicine keeps people close to one another, conscious of their environment, and physically strong.

Besides all that, popular medicine is proof that a group of people can be self-sufficient.

Bárbara: The *jíbara* race is a strong one. But strength and endurance have been chipped away on both physical and ideological levels.

Cleo: I've seen it perpetrated through the educational system. As a child, I studied from books which pushed the idea that the old *jíbara* culture should be destroyed and replaced by the modern culture. Part of that was reflected in the idea that the only "real" medicine comes in the form of pills and injections.

M: In general, I think people are so used to equating price with quality that they find it hard to believe that something that's free, that comes right out of the ground as a kind of gift, could possibly have as much value as something expensive, especially something expensive that comes from a far away, romanticized place.

Bárbara: Yes, but today, Puerto Rican people are going to these very expensive and exclusive health food stores to see what they can learn about their health, and they're finding—in classy little jars for ridiculously high prices—the very same herbs that their grandmothers used to give them. That's helping to open people's eyes a bit. They realize, "Hey, this is my grandmother's own medicine they're selling to us as if it were something new. We had this medicine first."

Cheo: The people of Puerto Rico aren't blind. We see the alcoholism, the abuse of drugs like cocaine and heroin. Not to mention the fact that so many people have had bad experiences with prescription drugs and unnecessary surgery. We recognize that we have lost something important, something that can still be recovered.

We all have to realize that popular medicine isn't just a matter of prescribing remedies. It's part of an entire culture, and it involves a respect for the land. It also involves helping to maintain people's health by advising them about diet and nutrition.

The *jíbaros* ground corn in a mill made of native stone, and they knew how to increase the calcium content of the corn by adding lime to the soil. The corn was then mixed with beans to complement the protein, and food like that gives people a tremendous strength. I've seen 70 and 80-year old men and women working more and harder than some of the young people I know. Because no matter how muscular and athletic young people today may be, they don't have the endurance of our old timers, the people of two, three, and four generations back. That has a lot to do with the way they lived, working every day close to the soil, and with their diet: locally grown whole grains, vegetables, *viandas*, and fruits.

Bárbara: On the large farms, they planted corn, onions, garlic, beans for the entire year, maybe even rice. Every afternoon or evening, they would grind the corn to be used for the next day's *surullos* (corn fritters stuffed with cheese or meat), which would be delivered to the men in the fields as they worked. Manure was used for fertilizer, to strengthen the plants. There was no need to use chemical products.

Of course there was a time of great poverty, when the people didn't have land or anything to plant on it. And there was a great deal of illness. But if traditional knowledge and practices had been supported, I think the world today would have a tremendous respect for the resources of Puerto Rico and for the strength and ingenuity of our people.

M: In closing, do you have a message for the people of Puerto Rico?

Bárbara: Yes. Let's remember with our grandparents. And if we don't have grandparents, let's find people who can talk to us, who can tell us stories of the old days, about the old ways, about the home remedies which were so convenient, wholesome, and effective.

The plants are still with us. With a bit of effort and investigation, people could rediscover many things which they've forgotten because of the deculturization process, because of social pressure to forget. Our old people are still alive.

Cheo: Let's learn all we can now because when we leave our health to the chemical companies, our sickness ends up benefitting them and we jeopardize our well-being with the side effects of dangerous drugs. We should become more conscious, try to recuperate the lost wisdom of our tradition. This will strengthen us as individuals and as a people.

Bárbara: I think there's a type of awakening going on. People are beginning to have more interest in knowing about their health and especially about medicinal plants because they know that their grandparents used them and they worked. And they still remember. Our tradition is alive in our folklore. It's under the rug right now, but it's very much alive.

Healing with Plants for Sixty Years

doña María and don Geño

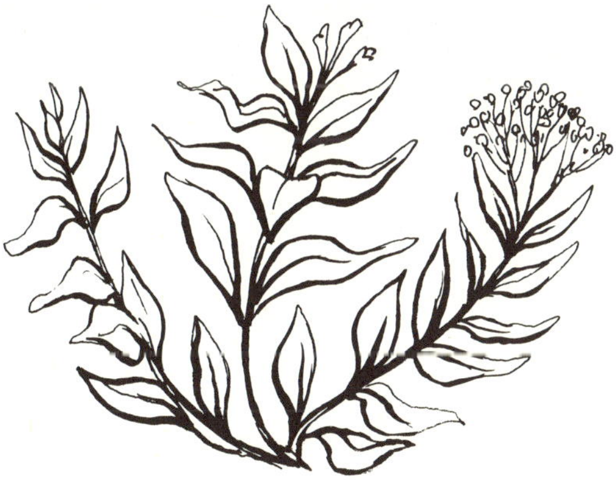

la salvia

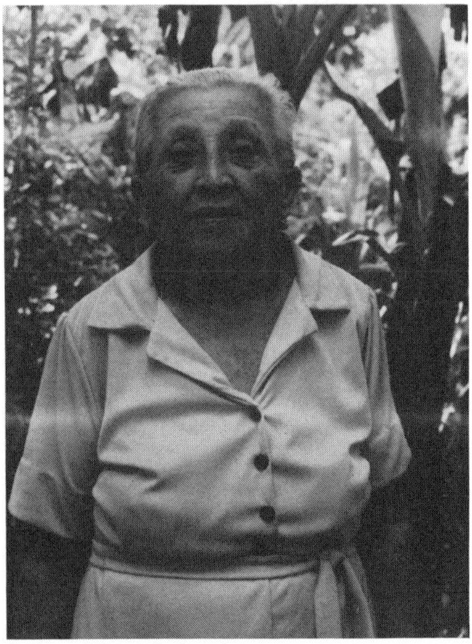

María Otero Collazo

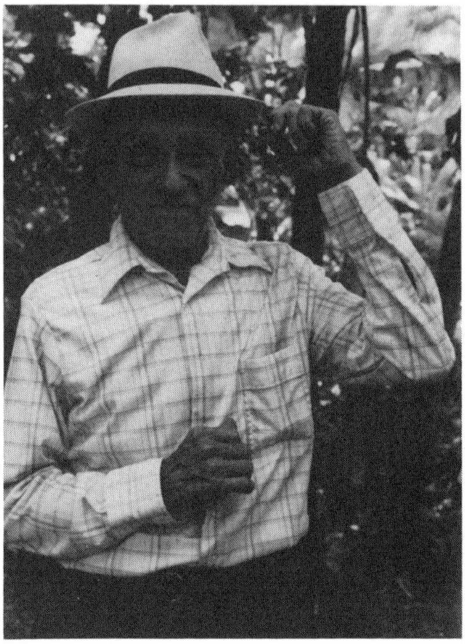

Eugenio Santiago Marrero

Healing with Plants for Sixty Years

doña María and don Geño

Doña María Otero Collazo de Santiago and don Eugenio Santiago Marrero were once the herbal physicians of their *barrio* in the countryside of Mayagüez. At age 75 and 84, they share a tremendous love for the natural world, and a wealth of experience using plants as medicine during their lifetime. Their knowledge comes from personal experience with the plants both through traditional family practices and through a willingness to experiment with the plants growing around them. Plants, along with spiritual practices such as prayer, are seen as optimum forms of medicine.

The following interview was held one May afternoon and evening in Morovis after a wonderful dinner prepared by doña María. Conversation ranged from the anecdotal to the encyplopedic as they talked of their experiences and shared their knowledge. Included here are not only remedies for health problems ranging from unrelenting fever to diabetes, women's infections, indigestion, headaches and lung problems, but also preventive medicines from purslane for avoiding bouts with intestinal worms to beef tallow for keeping the hands hardened when doing rough manual labor. Noteworthy too, are the uses of "*Agua Maravillosa*" (astringent witch hazel solution) for internal pain and removing blood stains from clothing. Clearly, they did not specialize.

In the world of doña María and don Eugenio, there are few rules, except those of good digestion. Don "Geño"—who was around to see Haley's comet the first time—enjoys his cigarettes and his daily shot of rum before dinner. He is proud to say that he has never had a headache, and according to the local hospital, his heart is "healthy as a child's."

Doña María makes it clear that everyone's system is different, that we all have different needs. Indeed, although their knowledge about plants is vast and they are aware of several properties of each plant they name, doña María's message seems to be that each episode of healing is an entirely unique experience. She doesn't follow recipes for her medicinal formulas (or for her cooking), but she knows what to do. The information she needs lives in her memory, and it is accessed through her dreams, through prayer, and through the intuitive act of preparing a remedy. She has even performed surgery when the occasion called for such a drastic measure.

Don Geño and doña María are living examples of a part of Puerto Rico's medical tradition—a tradition not only of information and practice, but also of attitude. For this couple, health is not just an absence of physical malaise; it takes root in a spirit of interdependence with nature, and faith in a God who is always found in nature. Healing is an every day experience, a sacred experience, widely accessible, and not without humor.

M: Doña María, you've spent a good part of your life working with plants as a way of healing. How did you learn about this?

María: In the old days, every mother brought up her kids, always telling them what was good for just about every condition. My mother always told me that *salvia* tea worked when a period was late, when there was some irregularity in a woman's cycle. And she'd also say, "Listen, after drinking that tea, you can't drink anything cold because it will give you cramps." So we learned as we grew, along with the years.

I'm always picking and "bottling" plants, preparing them as medicine. That's because the way to cure yourself is to start trying things and see how you feel afterwards. If you use the plants, you'll learn which ones are good for you.

My daughter, in this world, plants are of the utmost importance.

Geño: Without them, what would we do? They supply us with food, with shelter, even oxygen!

M: Don Geño, what kind of experience do you have with plants?

Geño: Well, I know them pretty well. I was born in 1903, almost yesterday (laughter), and I've always been a farmer. I like medicinal plants. In fact, I used to dedicate myself to working with them. I even used to prescribe for people; I would tell them how certain plants could be used as their medicine. And every time I get sick, I cure myself with plants. For instance, I take a strong tea of *poleo* when I get the flu or a bad cold. Sometimes, *los guarapos* work better than what a doctor might give you!

So I still go along planting herbs, although I do it less now that I'm old. It's a lot of work to condition the soil and keep all the different kinds of plants in their place. You have to fertilize them too, with cured cow and horse manure.

María: I also give the plants leftovers like potato skins and coffee grinds. The bitterness and acid of the coffee kills harmful microbes in the soil.

Geño: But animal fertilizer and food leftovers should be put in one place until it all cures and becomes compost, just like earth itself.

M: Can you talk about some of the medicinal plants you've used over the years?

Geño: In Mayagüez, in Villa Angélica, there was a famous *anacagüita* tree, which looked like a *ceiba*. The *anacagüita* gives a lot of flowers which are good for making *guarapo* for cold and flu. Plenty of people went there to look for the leaves. Yes, plants have always been people's medicine.

María: Sweet verbena (*yerba dulce*) has helped me a lot. First you boil it and then you put it in the refrigerator and drink it. The root is good for the stomach and for diabetes, too, because although it tastes very sweet, it has no sugar.

Geño: You can also just eat the leaf whenever you pass by the plant, or you can put the leaves in salad.

María: Two years ago, I tested positive five different times for diabetes. They put me on a special diet, but I still tested positive. So I started drinking sweet verbena boiled up with a pinch of yellow allamanda (*canario amarillo*) every day. Now, thank God, I've had more tests, and they can't find diabetes anywhere.

Cundeamor, which is very bitter, is also really good for diabetes. I boil the leaves up with the leaves of sweet verbena and it comes out like a *maví*. Actually, it's not so great tasting, but it's not too bad, cold. Just take a cup a day, right from the fridge.

I also had high blood pressure, and honey, they prescribed a mountain of pills! But the pills made me itch all over so I threw them out. Now I use passion fruit (*la parcha*). I just cut off the top and suck it and, holy cure that it is, I've had a bunch of tests done and I'm just fine!

So if they tell you you're about to die, well (laughter) . . .

Geño: If you live with *la doña,* you might be able to live at least 60 more years (laughter). Lord have mercy! Since I married her, we've spent so much time running up and down seeing and prescribing and curing without charging a penny. Sometimes we'd be called at nightfall, and we wouldn't get home till ten or eleven in the morning the next day. We traveled all over the countryside on foot, and everywhere we went, the plants that we needed were growing right where we happened to be.

M: Can you talk about some of the successes you've had?

Geño: I'd like to tell about something that happened in Mayagüez to a young girl, Panchita. She worked in the factory with *la doña.* Like everyone else, the youngster had to have her chest examined for tuberculosis. She had a flu at the time, so she was in no condition to be examined, but she had to go. And when they checked her, they found a spot on her lungs. So they laid her off and told her to go to the sanatorium, that she couldn't work any more. When she heard that, she started crying, and María saw her and asked her what was wrong. Panchita told her what had happened, and María said, "Don't worry. That little spot is nothing. I'm going to make you some medicine. I need a one gallon bottle, and the following plants, and I promise that by the time you've drunk half of what I prepare, you'll pass any lung test they can give you.

Panchita took the medicine every day, and when she was

almost finished, she went for another exam, and they didn't find a thing. She was in good health, and she never suffered from a lung problem again.

M: Do you remember the recipe?

María: Of course. I've used it so many times! Starting with the pharmacy: a four oz. bottle of each of the seven "syrups" (*los siete jarabes*) including *ipecacuana* syrup, chicory (*achicoria*) syrup, cocillana syrup (*jarabe pectoral*), balsam (*tolú*) syrup, star anise (*anís de estrella*), anise seed (*anís de grano*) and witch hazel solution (*Agua Maravillosa*). Then you peel three fat aloe vera (*sábila*) leaves and add all of the inside gelatin. Then juice large quantities of both watercress (*berro*) and *poleo*, and add some almond or cooking oil and some honey. Finally, you have to add a little rum or anisette in order to preserve it. When you're done, you should have a gallon of liquid. You don't have to cook it, but you do have to let it sit in the refrigerator for five or six days so that it really becomes one big syrup. Then drink it over a week's time or so. I'm telling you, my friend, many people have been cured with this formula!

M: Do you think that the ability to work with plants is a gift which only certain people have?

Geño: I think certain people have the blessing of being born to do that sort of work. They somehow know what to do.

M: I notice that you don't use any kind of recipe book as a source of remedies.

María: No, I invent everything. That's how it is when you're born to do something. I do everything from my head. And it's the same in the kitchen. You'll never find a cookbook around, although I can prepare all kinds of food. Once I try something and like it, I don't forget how I made it. I don't have to be tasting all the time. Thanks to God, I still have a clear mind.

And there's medicine in the kitchen, you know. Take cooking oil, for instance. It's a simple thing, but it's tremendous. Almost no-one believes in it anymore, but if you have a bad chest problem, take a tablespoon of cooking oil every morning, and the problem is eliminated little by little. The oil simply cleans out your chest. Nowadays everyone believes in fans and air conditioners, but they just weaken you.

Geño: There are lots of things the people of today don't know about. For example, hardly anyone uses tallow sticks (*sebo Flandes*) these days.

María: When someone has a fever, you take two pieces of tissue paper (the wrapping kind) just big enough to cover the soles of the person's feet. Actually they should be a little big so that when you put socks on, the paper can fold around the feet. Rub the *sebo Flandes* into the paper. Then take a little salt, a little sugar, and roll a bottle over it until it's ground up fine. Then you put that powder on top of the paper covered with tallow and sprinkle some cooking oil on top of all that.

Next, you prepare a bandage for the person's forehead the very same way. Exactly the same. Then you light a candle and use it to warm the bandage (don't put it too close, of course), and put the bandage on the person's head. Do the same with the paper soles, and put them on the soles of the person's feet. Finally, you put on some warm socks, and the person goes to sleep

The person should sleep as much as s/he wants and you don't take off those little paper soles until the next day. That's the remedy for stubborn fevers that simply won't go down. It always works!

Geño: Working people use tallow sticks too. Someone who does manual labor will use it to toughen up his hands. It heals and protects the skin. After work, you take a bath, and rub on some *sebo Flandes*. The next day, your hands are as hard as iron. It's the best there is!

When I started doing manual labor, they put me to work with metal shafts, and my hands were destroyed. By the end of the day, they were dripping with blood. But I'm the type to never say "I can't go on," so I kept working. Then an older gentleman told me about rubbing some *sebo Flandes* into my hands for protection. As soon as I left work, I bought five little tallow sticks for a penny a piece. That night, I took one and rubbed it into my hands. The next day my hands were dry and strong, and I kept working with no problem. Every day after work I put some more on my hands, and after that, nothing hurt them.

María: And he's telling you from experience. He's tried it, just as I've tried all the things I've told you about.

Geño: You can also use it when someone has a flu or chest cold. Just rub it into a porous piece of cloth and apply the cloth to the person's chest, or put the *sebo Flandes* directly onto the skin and then cover it up with cloth. I've seen it done both ways.

María: Another way of dealing with the same problem is by first rubbing the chest with a cloth soaked in *alcoholado* (herbs infused in alcoholic solution). Then you put plenty of *numoticina* (a rubefacient used in chest plasters) on top of that cloth with some camphorated oil (*aceite alcanforado*). That's your poultice, which must be worn, covered with cotton. Then you cover the poultice and cotton with a shirt and wait until the person begins to sweat and sweat. All the while, the person is breathing hard to get that air, the vapor of the medicine. That's how I've cured many a chest cold.

Of course, *la curía* is also very good for colds, and so is *la clavellina*, but only the yellow kind. White *clavellina* is just for show.

M: Your son-in-law told me that when Alma had a bronchial infection, her lungs were badly congested, and you helped her a lot.

María: When I took that girl in she was seven months old, and she weighed seven pounds, fourteen ounces. My word, her stomach was swollen, and if you gave her a bottle of milk, the milk would come out through her nose instead of going down into her stomach. Her little legs were bent backwards, completely immobile. And she was so weak, she could hardly cry. Geño said, "*Ay bendito*, we'll have to bury her in a few days. And I said, "Don't worry. She'll get better if God wills it, and God is so very great."

The next day I sent for a little bottle of castor oil, a dollar's worth of lime phosphate, and *Elixir* as a solvent. The medicine arrived that night. I gave her a little spoonful of the castor oil, and she slept through the night quietly, happily. The next day, she didn't even stir, and I thought she might be dying.

At six o clock in the evening, I was totally involved in praying to the Virgin Mary when suddenly I was moved to pick the baby up and hold her. At that moment, her little intestines started working. "Geño," I called. "The girl is alive and she's moving her bowels!" My lord, she emptied herself out completely. She had been fed rice water without salt, and that caused her whole stomach to seize up with a terrible indigestion and blockage.

I stayed up all night with her, giving her herb teas with

milk, feeding her. And the next day she woke up happy. Those remedies had done their work.

Afterwards, I asked permission from an aunt of mine to fish in the stream that ran by her house. "Sure," she said. "Come by whenever you like." So I went fishing at seven in the morning, when most of the creatures were still asleep, and I found a little fresh water crab (*buruquena*), and I rubbed parts of it on the soles of the baby's feet in the sign of a cross. Then I took a special plant called traveller's joy (*afilerillo*). I boiled it, added a little rum as a preservative, and rubbed it into her knees and legs. And look at how strong she walks now!

Then, when she was older, she got that terrible chest condition, and I began to prepare the same remedy I had made for Panchita: the seven syrups, plant juices, oil, honey and alcohol. I gave that to her morning and night. By the time she was scheduled for her operation, there was nothing wrong with her. The doctor said it was a miracle, that her lungs were completely clean. He wanted to know who had cured her.

Geño: He even took a jar of the remedy with him. Said he was going to study it! (laughter)

M: You mentioned using rum to preserve your remedies. In the northern U.S., we prepare many remedies in alcohol because, since we have such a long cold season, we often need a plant when it's not available. Plus it's much easier for people working outside of the home to take a few drops of tincture than it is to boil up a plant. Can you talk more about using alcohol in preparing medicines here in Puerto Rico?

Geño: Yes, we preserve medicines with alcohol, and I'll tell you something. We all need a little alcohol. Not to get drunk on, but to use. Our bodies need a little bit of everything, and a little rum can be used by the body like medicine. It also helps to sustain you sometimes while you work. But only up to two shots! Any more will do more harm than good.

María: Sometimes we add witch hazel solution to a remedy, and that has alcohol in it. Witch hazel solution is the greatest thing for cleaning mucus out of the lungs. It's also great for blood-stained clothing. Throw your clothes in to wash with a bottle of witch hazel and the blood comes right out.

Geño: Witch hazel is excellent for any internal pain you might have. But there are other things for pain, too. For instance, there are therapeutic baths that treat pain and illness. Several plants—such as eucalyptus (*eucalipto*) and bitter orange leaves (*el naranjo*)—serve for both internal and external use, for *guarapo* and for baths. Then there are plants which are used exclusively for baths. *Santa María* is one of them. It's only used externally, as far as I know.

M: How do you prepare a bath?

Geño: We fill a big vat with water, and throw in all the plants once the water boils. Now it's not taking a bath, exactly; it's more like having a bath poured over you. Because you can't use soap. You have to be clean already before receiving it. And you can't just splash the water every which place, either. You have to start at the top, at the head, and cover the entire body. That's how you receive the bath. Afterwards, you don't wash with soap, ever.

María: For a good bath, you pick roses and all the other flowers that are around, along with the leaves of avocado (*aguacate*), mango, coffee (*café*), and more. You boil them all up in a pot as if you were making a big soup. Then you leave it for the next day or at least a few hours, because if it's too hot you could get a muscle cramp. Then after you've taken a bath for cleanliness, get into the tub and receive the stream of water as it is poured down over you from your head to your feet. *Higuillo oloroso* is very good for baths.

Geño: *La doña* has cured me a number of times using baths and just about everything else.

María: I've had plenty of challenges, plenty of tests. About 60 years ago, he was in bed for five months straight, and the whole time he was delirious. If you could have seen him! He couldn't stop moving around in the bed, he didn't recognize anyone, and no one could understand what he was saying. I was with him all the time. The doctor came too, two or three times a day, but finally he gave up and said, "Bring this dead man to the sanatorium." The only medicines he gave after that were tranquilizers, by injection, so that Geño might die peacefully.

One night, Geño began screaming in a frightening way. I did my best to feed him. I boiled a chicken and some beef along with some baby doves. I added broadleaf coriander (*recao*), common plantain leaves (*llantén*), and mashed, green banana cakes (*tostones*). Then I strained the whole thing so he could drink it as if it were juice. The poor thing, he was all curled up like a little baby, and he tried to drink, but he couldn't stop the screaming; it went on all night long.

The next night, he held on to his bladder, and how he screamed! Everyone in the house was just waiting for him to die. They'd even bought the funeral candles. But at six in the evening I decided to do something. I went to a neighbor's house and asked, "Moncho, you have kids; do you have one of those syringes for the ears?" He did. So I went into the garden and gathered a bunch of *paletaria,* which I washed, boiled up and strained. Next I got rid of everyone who was in the room with him. I said, "Let me be alone with him for a while," and they all went into the living room.

I wrapped his penis in cloth, and I filled the syringe with the *paletaria* I'd prepared. Then I held him as I emptied the syringe into the urinary opening. The liquid stayed inside, and he was calm.

I emptied three syringes, and when I put a little basin out for him, there was a noise, and everything came out again, along with lots of blood. And that was the blessed cure. He has never suffered again with any kind of bladder or kidney problem.

M: How did you get the idea to do that?

María: I knew that *paletaria* was a good treatment for the bladder, and since it was originally a urinary problem, it seemed natural to work with it directly that way. I never had to give him any other treatment.

M: I've never heard of anyone using that method for men, but in the United States, women use similar "direct" methods. For vaginal infections caused by bacteria, for instance, we use suppositories of garlic or other natural antiseptic medicines. For other types of infections we do internal washes or use tampons soaked in herbal formulas.

María: *Campana* is very good for women's inflammations and infections. It makes a very good douche solution, but it's hardly planted any more because it's been abused as a drug.

And there are ways to deal with bladder problems orally. For instance, the leaves of mallow (*malva*) and black nightshade (*mata gallina*) can be boiled up together, and you can add some *paletaria* and spineless (*tuna*) cactus too. You should take the remedy at least every day, and always at night. It usually cures completely, but you have to continue with the remedy for a while before it really takes effect.

Geño: She cured me of another problem during that same illness. I have a scar on my back to prove it.

María: He was just a pile of bones, lying in that bed! I spent lots of time washing him. The problem was that he was always lying face up, and there was a great deal of friction with the sheets against his back, not only from his own restless movements in the bed, but from my pushing him this way and that when I tried to bathe him on one side, then the other, and then dry him. Of course, as he rubbed, his skin got all scratched up.

One morning I woke up and I saw a bunch of little worms or maggots moving around in his bed. And since everything was so clean, I couldn't figure out where they were coming from. So I started looking, and I saw that it was his back, which was all burned from the friction. There were bedsores, and that's where the little creatures were coming from.

At nightfall, when things were quiet, I calmly boiled some scissors. My mother in law asked me, "María, what are you doing?" And I said, "Oh I'm just making some tea."

Then I took some cotton and began to cut the area in his back which had maggots. There was a sort of hollow spot where everything was rotten, so I had to cut through that flesh, and I left it sunken in. The only disinfectant we had in the house at the time was boric acid, so I washed it well with a boric acid solution and kept quiet about what I'd done.

Geño: Just in case she'd killed me! (laughter)

María: The next day, I washed it again with boric acid and I applied a special pomade. Then I told my mother-in-law what I had done. "You're going to kill that poor man," she said.

And I said, "But if he's going to die anyway, he's going to die."

Geño: And look at how well it turned out. (*Don Geño shows off his "map" of scars.*)

M: Now I know you didn't learn to perform surgery from your mother! (laughter)

In the tradition of healing that I've studied, it's said that there are no rules, that each situation is completely unique, and that our intuition is a rich source of information. In the case you've just described, you received information, perhaps through prayer, and responded to a unique situation in a non-conventional but perfect way.

María: Yes, I've received a great deal of information through prayer and also through my dreams.

Back in Mayagüez, we knew a man who was always sick with something or other. He suffered from terrible fevers and nerve-wracking headaches. He was a widower, and I felt sorry for him because he didn't have anyone else to talk to. He came over to our house a lot.

Well, one night I dreamed I added salt to some ashes of *madera del pais* (the wood of an endemic tree that was commonly used to cook with), and put that mixture in hot water. Then I put a bandage soaked in that mixture on the man's forehead, and put his legs, from his knees down, into the bucket with the water, ashes and salt. The important thing was that both the water on his legs and the bandage on his forehead were really hot. Hot salt water with ashes.

That's what I dreamed, and I tried it the next day. He had a fever and a headache that was driving him crazy. It was as if all the blood in his body had gone to his head. Well, blessed be!

The remedy I'd dreamed about brought that blood down. He felt just fine afterwards, and calm.

Geño: You can talk about dreams, and you can talk about faith. After the Virgin appeared at the well in Sábana Grande* thirty years back, sick people started going, and they still fill up the chapel! People go in wheelchairs and walk out without any help at all.

We had a neighbor who was paralyzed with a serious condition that the doctors considered to be incurable. She'd been ill for nine years but one day she decided to visit the well at Sábana Grande. And when she arrived in her little cart, she was healed. She simply stood up and told the woman who cared for her, "I want to walk back," and she did. So at times, it's faith that does the healing, and not the medicine itself. It's the faith that you have in the food or in the water or in the plant. You should see that shrine with all the writings of people who have been cured, and all the crutches that have been left there. There have been so many miracles!

M: Today so many people live in cities where it's easy to forget about the every-day miracle of life-giving plants. I'd like to hear more about your own relationship with the earth.

Geño: Very simply, plants are the best medicine, better than anything a doctor can prescribe. It's hard to understand, but most doctors today don't know a thing about plants.

I believe in plants. If I take some leaves for a *guarapo*, I look for certain properties. For instance, I'll look for a plant that's heating, or one that's cooling, which is good for when you've got a flu caused by heat. If your illness is caused by cold, you'd never administer a cooling remedy; that would only make the person sicker.

María: *El cundeamor* is a heating plant.

Geño: It can even burn you!

María: The other day, one of our neighbors here got sick, poor thing. They took her to the hospital and her legs were a real mess with all the itching. In fact, she was taking injections because she just couldn't stop scratching her legs, and water was oozing out.

I went to see her and asked, "Can I prepare you a wash for your legs?" And she said, "Why not, my love? But you should know that I'm almost dead."

I came and boiled up two gallons of *cundeamor*, which she applied and also drank. Blessed cure! The itching disappeared and she was healed. Because *cundeamor* is bitter, and it's warming.

So the doctor came and asked, "What in the world did you put on that?" She said, "A neighbor did me the favor with *cundeamor*. And he said, "Don't tell me that *cundeamor* is medicine!" But it certainly is.

And listen, the palma Christi or castor bean plant (*higuereta*) is heating.

Geño: It's *very* heating, and it's laxative, too.

María: It's good for when a woman gives birth and part of the placenta remains inside. A sitz bath of palma Christi leaves boiled up will help to clean her out. Palma Christi is also good for animals who give birth and get stuck with the placenta.

Another form of using the palma Christi is to make a little necklace of its cut, hollow leaf stems. You just break the leaf stems up, string them and put them on the person's body. It's good for any type of inflammation.

Geño: If you use the castor bean plant on the cows when milk balls form in their udders, they'll give more milk. You simply take the plant and boil it in a big tub. Then, after it's boiled long enough so that the water has taken on the color of the leaves, you skim off the foam. The next day, when you go to the cows in the morning, you take that liquid, and with the very same leaves you boiled, you wash the udder completely, and with lots of strength. You do this two or three times a day, and you'll see the milk balls disappear. She'll get better soon and I guarantee, she'll start giving more milk.

M: I'm really interested in learning more about which plants are hot, which are cold, and the difference between the two kinds of plants.

Geño: *Poleo* is hot. It's great for chest colds. Aloe is hot. It's also very good for the chest, and so is *malá*, which works in a similar way.

The root of *yerba guinea* is hot. On the other hand, mallow (*malva*) is cool, *guanábana* leaf is cooling, black nightshade (*mata gallina*) is cooling.

Caribbean vervain (*verbena*) is hot, warming.

María: For the stomach, and for fevers.

GENIO: Snake plant (*el chucho*) is hot.

María: Snake plant root is really good for a bad cough, even a desperate case of the whooping cough. You just boil the grated root up with water or with coconut water and take it as needed.

Geño: Bitter orange leaves are cooling.

María: They're really the best thing for your nerves.

Geño: And everyone knows that *paletaria*, *cohitre blanco* and purslane (*verdolaga*) are cooling.

María: Purslane can be given to children to avoid their getting worms.

Geño: You boil it up and give it to them in tea, like wormseed (*pazote*). Wormseed is best, but it stinks so badly that you have to hold your nose in order to drink it. That's the bad part. But if you have worms, it will make them leave your body in droves!

María: What a stink!

Geño: Sometimes the herbs that are the worst to take get the best results. Wormseed is the best thing in the world for worms because it actually breaks them up into pieces before it expels them.

M: That reminds me of valerian (*valeriana*), which also has a terrible smell. But it's great for helping you sleep or even just relax when you're very anxious or under a lot of stress.

María: They sell valerian tincture in drops now at the drug store. You put a few drops in water for your nerves.

Geño: Listen, the leaves and flowers of coffee senna (*hedionda*) are good for gas. They make a great cure mixed in a *guarapo* with anise seeds.

And you can use coffee senna seeds to make a type of coffee. Just toast them, but keep the flame low so they don't burn. Then boil them up. Delicious! I'd say that coffee senna is hot.

María: Caribbean vervain (*verbena*) root is very good for indigestion. When one has eaten too much, or when one has eaten something disagreeable, a good *guarapo* of vervain gets rid of the discomfort, and it makes a good gargle, too.

Geño: Vervain is hot, but you have to be able to recognize the medicinal vervain, which has a stalk that grows straight up above the main plant, and bears a little purple flower. The other vervain looks something like the real thing, but it's no good for medicine.

Wild jessamine (*yapaná*) is also hot and we use it in guarapo for colds, to get rid of any coldness in the body, and related conditions.

María: Plantain (*llantén*) is good for hemorrhage, and boiled up with black nightshade, it's a good treatment for stomach ulcers.

Geño: Plantain leaves and roots are hot. And lemon grass is hot.

María: Lemon grass tea is great for fevers.

Geño: All ginger (*jengibre*) is hot. Sweet, native ginger (*jengibre dulce*) is good for teas, and bitter ginger (*jengibre amargo*), grated and boiled in oil, is good for massages.

María: Bitter ginger in oil is great rubbed into arthritic joints. Sweet ginger with milk will help you to get rid of a bad cold in your chest. And sweet ginger with coconut milk tastes wonderful!

Geño: Ginger is good for so many things. If you're making coconut candy and you put in a little sweet ginger, those treats will have a phenomenal taste, while without the ginger, they won't taste like anything. You can add a bit of ground ginger to almost anything, even to your regular cooking and baking flour. It gives everything a good flavor.

Tuatúa is neither hot nor cold, but I'd say that it *is* warming.

María: You want to pull the leaf down off the stalk if you want your body to get rid of waste from the bottom (laughter). Pull it up if you want to throw up.

Geño: *Tártago* is like that. Take three leaves and pull them upward. Drink a tea of those leaves, and you'll throw up because you pulled them upward. A tea of leaves pulled downward will get rid of your nausea. I've never done it, but all the old people of my day said it worked. I think it has to do with the sap of the plant being released more when you pull it one way or the other. I'd say *tártago* is a hot plant.

María: Once this guy here ate something that gave him bad indigestion and diarrhea. He was sick for days, and he was starting to look like a skeleton. He didn't want any medicine, but I finally told him, "Look, either you take this medicine or I'll pour it over your head." Well I boiled up three leaves of *tártago*, and then with some cooking oil, I began rubbing his stomach gently in the form of a cross, pushing down and pushing cross-wise, too. Then I added a bit of salt and sugar to the tea I'd made, and he drank it. Miracle cure! He vomited what was in his stomach almost immediately, and the next day his stomach was so strong that he could have eaten a plate full of rocks!

Geño: Have some of this eucalyptus (*eucalipto*). It's really hot, and it's good for colds, just like *anacagüita*.

María: *El cariaquillo* is also very good for colds.

M: I've heard that the leaves and stems of native lentils (*gandul*) are effective for diabetes.

María: Yes, and they're quite bitter.

Geño: I've heard people say that the native lentil plant is cooling, but I'd say it's hot.

María: Mugwort (*altamisa*) is good for baths.

Geño: It's hot.

María: Yellow elder (*saúco amarillo*) is hot. It's for a cold in the chest.

Geño: There are two kinds of elder, you know. The yellow elder is better than the white.

María: Spineless tuna cactus is cool, and it's good for the kidneys.

Geño: Basil (*albahaca*) is cooling, and it gives a good smell to your food. It's also good for baths and for alcohol rubs. You add it to an alcohol solution (*alcoholado*), and when you have body pains, you give yourself a rub with it.

María: Besides that, it makes a good *guarapo*, and basil's tiny seeds can be put into the inside corners of the eyes, very gently, so that they don't irritate. Left a little while there, they'll clear your vision. The seeds seem to attract anything that shouldn't be in the eyes.

Geño: Red mint (*yerba buena*) is good and cooling for the stomach, and *cohitre blanco* is another cooling plant. The leaves of bay rum (*la malagueta*) and *salvia* are heating. And *ipecacuana* is one of the most effective of the hot herbs. It's tremendous.

María: We used to take three little pieces of *ipecacuana* and put them in a glass of water. That was boiled up, and it helped you to vomit up all the phlegm you might have in your chest. And *malá* is like aloe; it's also good for chest problems. *La gran señora* is a hot herb that can be harvested in Mayagüez, but it's nowhere to be found around here. A *guarapo* of *gran señora* is great for fever; in fact, it's the best treatment if you have a flu with high fever, alternating hot and cold.

And rosemary (*romero*) is a hot herb. They used to say that it was good for the memory, you know. But I've always had a good memory, so I've never used it for that.

M: What do you do to treat boils and other small growths?

María: Do you know about "the weed that even the goats won't eat?" Garlic weed (*el anamú*) has a strong smell, but it used to be really popular as a hot compress for growths that wouldn't burst open. And it was used in the form of a tea when a woman didn't want to have children. It's abortive.

Geño: Almost any leaf heated up can be used to break open a boil or tumorous growth, because it's the heat, actually, that does the work. You can use hot leaves or hot cloths—even a cooked egg! And as the growth opens up with the heat, you feel a tremendous relief.

M: What's that plant over there?

Geño: *Escobilla*. Before it flowers, it makes a lather, and you can actually wash with it. They used to use it to bathe the horses, and even to wash dishes.

María: It's good for skin rashes, and it's great for washing little children when their sensitive skin gets irritated. You can bathe the tiniest baby with it.

And annato (*achiote*) is good when someone has a painful inflammation. You put the leaf on top of the inflammation, and it's soothed. It's especially good for toothache.

Geño: Not to mention for headaches. You can rub the leaf with cooking oil and stick it on to your forehead. If it's doing the job, the leaf will dry out and break up until it's powder. It just draws the heat right out of you. If it stays wet and slides around, it's simply not the remedy you need.

María: Marjoram (*mejorana*) is good for the ears. When you have an ear ache, you warm up the leaf and chop it up until the juice seeps out of the leaf. Pick up that warm juice with a pad of cotton and squeeze it into the ear. Then cover it with the cotton.

Geño: In my opinion, arrowroot (*maranta*) is the greatest, the starchy part. Down by my old house, where we had the farm, there was so much arrowroot. It's like *yautía*. Actually, the plant looks like a little yam, and when you harvest it, you take the little egg-like roots, and *¡ave María!* are they good in stew. I could win a contest eating them!

Then for medicine, you just had to grate them and take the starch. The starch can also be used as baby powder to alleviate heat rash beneath kids' diapers.

María: Women also used arrowroot powder after bathing for other kinds of irritations. And that reminds me, rue is useful for uterine problems. So is broadleaf coriander (*culantro del monte*), which is great for high blood presure.

Geño: And you can add broadleaf coriander to almost any medicinal tea.

María: Also, burnt *bálsamo* is tremendous. The ashes of that bush will cure any wound. Monche's son's leg was really a mess, but he cured it with the ashes of *bálsamo*—the kind that grows high and is very leafy.

Oyster plant (*sanguinaria*) is good for hemorrhage, and even for heart irregularities. You can boil a little or just make a tisane, adding some to cold water and leaving it for a day. But you've got to drink it sparingly; don't take too much of it, ever. It's also a fine remedy if you've been bruised. You can chop or mash it up and put it on top of the bruise with a little salt, as a poultice. That's a good treatment.

Geño: Speaking of the heart, there's *corazón*, which is very good after someone has a heart attack. The leaf is warmed up and placed over the heart. Taken in medicinal teas it also prevents further attacks.

María: There are so many herbs that can be boiled and served as medicinal tea, or cold from the refrigerator like ice water or lemonade: lemon grass, bitter orange leaves, *curía* and so many more can be used like that.

Geño: You know, though I'm 84 years old, I have never once had a headache. Never in my life. And I don't think I'll have one in the next few years before I die either. In fact, I don't have any pains at all! Being old isn't painful for me. But people are always bothering me about my cigarettes, that I'm going to die, that they'll give me cancer. I tell them, "I've been smoking for almost 75 years, since I was ten years old. Smoking and drinking rum too, sometimes at the same time, losing nights of sleep, working day after day, and I'm alive! I'm just fine!

Five years ago I was out milking the cows at six in the morning, and all of a sudden, one of the cows knocked me over and I fell onto a big rock. I lay there unconscious for almost an hour. When I came to, I was all bruised and covered in blood. In fact, I was swallowing my own blood, but I did manage to drag myself home. My daughter wanted me to go to the doctor's office, but I didn't want to go. I said, "No. There's nothing wrong." But a few days later when I went to the bathroom, it could be that my eyes played a trick on me, but it seemed that I was bleeding a little bit. So I went to San Pablo Hospital, and I stayed there for seven days.

They did every kind of test on me, with all their fancy new equipment. I half expected them to put a periscope up my elbow so they could see what was up there. But they couldn't find any problem at all. Finally they let me go home and told me to come back in a week for another check up.

So I went back to see the doctor, and he gave me a check up. Afterwards, he asked me, "So you smoke?" I said, "Of course I smoke." He said, "And your chest; is there anything wrong with your chest?" So I said, "Well, once in a while I cough, but only what's normal." And he checked me out all over again and couldn't find anything wrong with me. He told me that my heart was like a child's. He said, "You're perfectly alright. You don't have any illness at all." That's when I told him I'd never even had a headache. He just looked at me, and you know what he said? He said I might just last another thirty years!

María: It's important to realize that everyone isn't the same. One person can smoke or drink something, and it does no harm at all, while if I do the very same thing, I'll be ready to die from it in no time at all.

For instance, I can't get away with drinking even a little bit of coffee. Not too long ago, I tried it for the millionth time. I was cold all over because I hadn't eaten well during the day—I simply had no appetite. Then at about 9:30 at night, I drank some coffee, and felt fine. But in the morning, I was so sick, so very sick, that I had to take a purgative.

Other people can drink coffee at any hour of the day or night and it does no harm at all. But even just the smell of coffee can make me sick.

Geño: Everyone is different, but I think that the way one eats is the most important thing. Not that you should only eat a little; you can eat all you want. But you should wait until it's time to eat. Because if you have a big lunch at twelve and you eat again at 1:30, you're interfering with the process of digestion. And if you keep on doing it, you're going to have trouble. Lots of trouble.

María: Eating too fast can give you gas. But if you're uncomfortable—or worse—after eating, there's anise, which is a heating remedy.

There's always a remedy for everything, you know. In this world, my daughter, plants are truly a wonder.

Don Geño passed away in November 1987, six months after having participated in this interview. He wasn't sick, nor was he in pain. He died of heart failure just minutes after having tended the animals, when he lay down to watch TV.

Passing It On

epilogue

In April of 1987, I went to Puerto Rico for the first time, but I was going home. Home to *arroz con gandules* and *bacalao con pana*, to *arroz con coco,* the rich flavor of bright yellow *apio*, and tall glasses of *refresco de guanábana.* Home to *la bendición* and holy week processions and plaster of Paris saints on bedroom altars. Home to the country sound of roosters at all hours of the day and night, and *bomba, plena* and *salsa* in the city streets and local buses. I went home to outdoor concerts of *le lo lai,* African rhythms, and Indian flute sounds all in one. To where hospitality said "family" everywhere I went. Home to where our elders and rural young people know and work with the healing power of plants, and to where the tiny *pitirre* attacks and wins battles with the bandit *guaraguao.* Home to where the wind, sun, tides and red earth are guardians of the past and sacraments of all possibility.

But I also went home to a country struggling under an economy based not upon the island's strengths (abundant fresh water, extremely fertile soil, small size, accessibility to diverse waterways and neighboring countries, capacity for solar, wind, sea and other types of safe, renewable energy generation) but on its "insufficiency" of resources. Home to where industrial pollution of soil and water represents a serious risk for large segments of the population. And I went home to a people challenged by the devaluation of their own rich culture of healing ways.

Earth and Spirit: Healing Lore and More from Puerto Rico is based upon the knowledge and generosity of people in Mayagüez, Las Marías, Morovis, Carolina, Orocovis, Loíza Aldea, Río Piedras, Caguas, Luquillo, and Fajardo. My investigation was limited to a six-week period, and even in such a short time I was able to glimpse a tremendous tradition of herbal medicine, spiritual healing, and connection with the land. But along with the exciting stories of healing successes, I was also told stories of disappeared species, the poisoning of earth and precious water tables, and the devaluation of elders' knowledge and experience by those who have learned that only modern pharmaceutical preparations can heal.

In Puerto Rico, traditional practices are rapidly disappearing, along with our elders. The tendency of outsiders (and those who internalize outsiders' values) to associate Puerto Rico's traditional medicine with ignorance, plus economic structures which have led to growing dependence upon non-indigenous products and practices, contribute to a devaluation and rejection of a tremendously useful system of human exchange and mutual aid.

In fact, this system represents far more than the healing of people and animals. One of the most important aspects of folk medicine is its basic dependence upon healthy natural surroundings. Traditional healing practices help to maintain the integrity of the natural world, and folk healers educate others about the environment through harvesting, planting and related lore. In this way, traditional healers are also ecologists, supporting the web of life shared by all species.

As we are confronted with the deterioriation of the earth's ozone layer—as well as crises such as the foreseeable end of petroleum supplies and the proliferation of deadly nuclear waste—more than ever, we need safe, renewable natural resources. For instance, we need biomass for alcohol to replace gasoline, natural rubber and fibers to replace those based on petrochemicals, green medicine to supplement and expand synthetic sources. For our own physical survival and the survival of generations to come, economic and social systems all over the world must prioritize the development of technologies and industries which are ecologically sound.

Yet—considering just one front of the problem—in the developing world, foreign debt forces countries to make way for capital-intensive but ecologically disastrous industries like petroleum exploration, cattle grazing, and lumbering. As a result, our precious tropical rain forests are being destroyed at a rate of 50-100 acres a minute.[1]

Tropical rain forests, though accounting for only 7% of the Earth's surface, provide habitat for 50%–80% of the world's plant and animal species. Utilizing carbon dioxide and producing a great deal of the world's oxygen, they give life in abundance and influence weather conditions throughout the world. (Recent weather pattern changes are partly blamed on accelerated deforestation since the 1950s.) At our present rate of destruction, 2/3 of Latin America's rain forests will have disappeared by the year 2000.

Dr. Oswaldo Guerrero, pharmacognosist at the University of Puerto Rico's College of Pharmacy comments, "We're losing one species of life each day and we really don't know what we're destroying." Of course, this is true not only in terms of plant life, but also in terms of indigenous knowledge and

[1] Rainforest Alliance 295 Madison Ave. Suite 1804, NYC, NY 10017 (212) 599-5060.

practices which are so closely related to the health and integrity of the area's ecology! He continues, "The same thing could be said of Puerto Rico, which has undergone a tremendous amount of development in a very short time."

Dr. Guerrero is focusing his own study on the island's endemic or native plants in danger of extinction. He explains that these plants promise to serve in diverse ways: from medicine to natural "diet" sweeteners to natural fibers, non-polluting insecticides, fertilizers, and other commercially valuable products. *Magnolia splendens*, for instance, is one of Puerto Rico's threatened species which has proven anti-bacterial action.

In 1989, over 25% of all drugs in the U.S. still consist of (as in the case of psillium seed) or contain plant material as principal active ingredients. And almost all other drugs are based on molecular models found in land and sea plants including fungi, and microbes. Throughout the western world, plants are, directly and indirectly, the source of almost all medical substances.

In Puerto Rico, 300 of the more than 3,000 species of plants growing on the island are already recognized by science as having positive medicinal action. And as evidenced throughout this book, many others hold the promise of medicinal, and perhaps commercial, value as well.

Although threatened by development and pollution, Puerto Rico's fertile hills and rain forest still offer a plethora of useful botanicals and related information. And since a large part of the medicine used in the western world is derived from tropical climates, the island could take on a greater role in leading the search for natural medicines.

While economic conditions may not now be ripe for full-scale commercial development, research and funding for exploratory projects involving the cultivation of medicinal plants and the manufacture of related products is certainly called for. Such valuable—and marketable—plants include *la parcha* (*Passiflora edulis*), which lowers blood pressure. (At present, most of the *parcha* consumed on the island is imported from the Dominican Republic, where agricultural wages are lower.) *Aloe vera* also holds tremendous promise as a money-making crop; it is currently used around the world as a purgative and tonic for the bronchial and digestive systems, a cosmetic for hair and skin, and first-rate ointment for burns and other conditions. Sesame might flourish as a tremendous source of high-quality cooking oil, and as a calcium-rich food. Small-scale studies have already shown that Puerto Rico's well known *cundeamor* (*Momordica charantia*) compares favorably as an anti-fungal agent with pharmaceutical preparations. And at least one study affirms popular knowledge that *baquiña cerrada* (*Lepianthus peltata*) is effective in dissolving kidney stones.

According to Dr. Esteban Núñez Meléndez, professor emeritus at the College of Pharmacy at the University of Puerto Rico and author of *Plantas medicinales de Puerto Rico*, "The Caribbean region has contributed many aromatic oils, which are used in creams, unguents and rubs absorbed by the skin." The aromatic essential oils offered by citrus trees and other plants abundant in Puerto Rico are highly valued throughout the hemisphere, not only for flavoring and scents in medicine and perfumes, but also in local anaesthetics and preservatives for emulsions. And the Caribbean periwinkle, *playera* (*Catharanthus roseus*), contains more than thirty alkaloids. Two of these are being used effectively against Hodgkin's disease, a lymphatic cancer[2].

[2] From *Plantas medicinales de Puerto Rico* by Dr. Esteban Nuñez Melendez, (Editorial de la Universidad de Puerto Rico, 1982) p. 77.

At the 1987 Congress of the North American Society of Phyto-chemistry held in Tampa, Florida, a study of 15 species selected from El Yunque—Puerto Rico's own tropical rain forest—found the plants to be precious enough so that "germ plasm repositories should be created for future preservation of the chemical potential of those plants."

In fact, as we face new diseases as well as growing numbers of new and drug-resistant strains of viruses and bacteria, the value of environments such as El Yunque can only grow.

Although synthesized drugs (drugs not based on actual plant material, but almost always based on the molecular structure of plant-based compounds) mean the most extensive profits for pharmaceutical companies[3], plants are of greater importance in the development of medicine today than ever before.

Dr. Mikhail Antoun, pharmacognosist at the University of Puerto Rico, emphasizes, "We're just beginning to learn about what nature has to offer. The only way to find the unimaginable, the truly new, is to work closely with nature, which is always full of surprises."

One of the greatest obstacles to the development and re-evaluation of natural medicine as a primary resource is the fact that Newtonian science[4] tends to equate the whole of a sub-

[3] According to the Herb Research Foundation's *Herbalgram* #15, winter 1988, a synthetic drug is patentable for 17 years, allowing pharmaceutical companies to recoup large profits on research & development investments and FDA-required tests for "new drug" status. (Approximately $120 million is spent on research and testing for each new drug.) Natural or "crude" drugs are not patentable, thus they offer less economic incentive.

[4] The term "Newtonian science" refers to the mechanistic science of pre-Einsteinian physics. Limited to a logical framework of cause and effect, Newtonian science simply can not explain or account for phenomena occuring in the atomic and subatomic realms.

Still working from a Newtonian base, "official" medical science depends stance with its molecular structure. Thus, two substances: the natural vitamin C found in a ripe, juicy orange, for instance and the synthesized vitamin found in a glass of artificially flavored Kool Aid are considered to be one and the same! The presence of a vital energy intrinsic in all things warmed by the sun, cooled by night breezes, wet by the rain and rooted in fertile earth is not measurable by standard scientific equipment; thus it is ignored.

Actually, some substances do defy the Newtonian equation. For instance, in its natural state, camphor is a solid compound. But its synthetic molecular "twin" is a liquid. Other natural compounds are either too unstable or just too difficult to synthesize. Thirty steps are involved in the process of synthesizing just one molecule of morphine. So poppies are still used as a source of morphine and other opium-derivatives. And in spite of millions of U.S. dollars invested in efforts to synthesize or even cultivate ergot (a fungus found naturally in grains—used to stimulate and accelerate labor in childbirth), science has found no substitute for the real thing.

Our bodies too respond to many "immeasurable" differences. As our ancestors have always known, and as the new physics[5]

---

for its validity, structure and progress upon repeatable phenomena as evidenced by replicated tests. Thus, synthesized products are favored, largely because their use eliminates variables which interfere in processes of repetition and testing or measurement.

[5] The "new physics," derived from Einstein's and other scientists' groundbreaking discoveries, recognizes (based upon observation of subatomic particles) the virtual impossibility of repetition as well as the constantly changing context of every reality, a context dependent upon physical and non- physical factors.

The new physics also recognizes what appears to be consciousness in even subatomic particles. In terms of healing, the implications are tremendous, is teaching us, nature is far more complex than we could ever have imagined. And the use of whole plants, especially those harvested in the wild, may offer many benefits not yet recognized by laboratory science.

Andrew Weil, M.D., Harvard graduate and author of *Health and Healing*, describes how a plant taken in its whole state may work more slowly than the pharmaceutical drugs derived from it, but that the use of the plant itself may be distinctly advantageous. He shows how the currently outmoded use of foxglove leaf (digitalis) allowed heart patients and their doctors to monitor excessive dosages through clear warning signals: nausea meant that a dose should be cut back, far before any damage was done to the heart. Today's isolated heart-stimulating compounds (digitoxin and digoxin) act quickly, and are invaluable in medical emergencies. But without the associate "non-active" compounds found in the crude plant form, there are no warning signs. Thus patients who could benefit from the slow acting and far safer, "whole" cardiac tonic are unecessarily exposed to the risk of iatrogenic (medicine-caused) arrhythmia and even heart attack. Coca (source of cocaine), ephedra (source of ephedrine—the asthma medicine often consumed in spray form) and willow bark (source of aspirin) are other examples of natural medicines whose isolated components are known to be addictive, carcino-

---

and validate the dignity of every healing approach, especially those which involve cooperation with one's environment and "communication" with disease on physical and non-physical levels.

genic or otherwise dangerous, but these dangers are neutralized by other compounds found in the plants themselves. As Dr. Weil asserts, "In general, isolated and refined drugs are much more toxic than their botanical sources. They also tend to produce effects of more rapid onset, greater intensity, and shorter duration. Sometimes they fail to reproduce desirable actions of plants they come from, and sometimes they lack natural safeguards present in those plants. They also lend themselves to methods of administration favoring abuse and toxicity."[6]

On the front of malaria treatment, the use of synthetic chloroquine has given rise to resistant strains of the offending mosquito (*Plasmodium falciparum*). According to the World Health Organization, in malaria-plagued parts of the world, infections are once again being treated with a combination of drugs now including quinine, which had been abandoned for many years in favor of synthetics.

Meanwhile, some antimicrobial synthetics, especially antibiotics, have been found to cause cell wall irregularities which may spawn new diseases. And it's becoming common knowledge that broad spectrum antibiotics—which (like pesticides) destroy useful, beneficial bacteria—are greatly responsible for the rise of the new (and largley non-diagnosed) overgrowth epidemic of the fungus, "candida." In the absence of beneficial bacteria, which normally live in the digestive tract, this fungus overpopulates, feeding upon sugar. It compromises the immune system, leaving its victims prone to illness, fatigue, depression and/or anxiety.

Ironically, while "Say NO to Drugs" is practically the official billboard of Puerto Rico's metropolitan areas, mile for mile

[6] Andrew Weil, M.D., *Health and Healing* (Boston: Houghton Mifflin Company, 1983) pp. 99–111.

there is perhaps more pharmaceutical industry on the island of Puerto Rico than anywhere else in the world. And while most of this industry produces for export, it's hard to ignore a relationship between the decline of the country's endemic medical culture and the rise of the petro-chemical-based pharmaceutical industry which, while offering obvious benefits including widespread employment, has also posed innumerable problems ranging from iatrogenic disease to local pollution, "legal" addiction, and cultural alienation.

On the bright side, at the University of Puerto Rico, pharmacological research is at a point of transition, sparked by a resurgence of interest in natural products, including folk culture's highly valued medicinal plants. University faculty members have proposed the development of an Institute of Natural Products, designed for the purpose of studying the plants of Puerto Rico. It would work closely with the Department of Natural Resources and—respecting the value of ethnobotany—with the people of Puerto Rico who know, love and use the plants found in their surroundings.

The proposed Institute, and all such endeavors to link laboratory science and empirical knowledge are not just "good ideas." They are bridges which will help us to create and maintain healthy environments for ourselves while enabling us to face acute medical problems and emergencies with greater understanding and efficiency. Such facilities lead the way toward the making of medical professionals who will value and prescribe not only products of today's pharmaceutical industry but also plant extracts, infusions, decoctions, tinctures, homeopathic preparations, and other forms of natural medicine in the effort to live up to their Hippocratic oath to "do no harm." Closing the gap between science and popular culture, these practices—at a time of ecological crisis—may even prove necessary for human survival.

On a personal level, each of us can find ways of working to protect and preserve the natural environment. And we can preserve the body of traditional medicine which exists through the lore alive in our own memories and the memories and practices of family members, neighbors and friends.

Valuing the land and valuing the tradition, recording the lore, learning to recognize the plants, using and cultivating them ourselves, encouraging others to do the same, we pass the tradition on. In this way we will create and practice medicine which truly heals not only our own minds and bodies, but also our relationship with the Earth. This is essential.

For the Earth is our past, and she is our future.

Healing Lore and More at a Glance

contributors

important terminology

a practical reference of herbal and related folklore

It has been a privilege to compile this practical reference, which represents a good deal of the knowledge and experience shared by the people I interviewed during April and May of 1987 in ten *pueblos* of Puerto Rico. This chapter includes recipes and lore from several non-published interviews as well as from interviews which have been included in this volume, but not in their entirety.

Important Terminology

In order to avoid repetitious phrasing, I've included definitions of terms used most frequently below:

TEA (also ***GUARAPO***): **not the three-minute teabag dip** we are so familiar with, the traditional, medicinal "tea" or *guarapo* of Puerto Rico is actually a decoction, made more or less (varying slightly from home to home) this way: To a litre of boiling water, add about a handful of well-rinsed, fresh plant material. (If using dried plants, use about 1/3 as much.) Then lower the heat, cover and simmer for about fifteen minutes, or until the water takes on a deep color, usually green. (Sitz baths and soaks are usually made according to similar proportions.)

According to several contributors, *guarapos* should be drunk a bit warm in the evening. During the day, they can be taken cold, like water. Some are prepared with honey.

MENORATIVA: A "tea" or *guarapo* made with more than three, and up to a dozen or more ingredients.

TISANE: A medicinal preparation prepared without heat. Usually, plant material steeped in cool water for hours, overnight, or days before consuming.

POULTICE: A damp pack, often made of plant material, placed upon an irritated or inflamed area of the body. Most poultices are used to soothe, increase circulation in an area, or draw out impurities and foreign matter.

BATH: Most baths and soaks are prepared like giant *guarapos*. Fresh plant material is added to a vat of water and boiled for 15–30 minutes before administering. See **Baths** on p. 181 for specific instructions.

ALCOHOLADO: An analgesic and cooling infusion of herbs in dilute rubbing alcohol, popular for rubdowns and massages. Sold commercially (Florida Water or *Agua Florida* is an example of a popular *alcoholado*), it is often improved upon by the personalized addition of herbs for specific purposes.

Each of us is unique, as are our physical conditions. No remedy described will be right for everyone, and each should be tried with intuitive wisdom (taking into account one's own needs and personal experience) and/or with the guidance of a person experienced in healing with plants.

The contributor of each remedy is identified by her or his initials, as follows:

AC:	Ana Clausells de Costoso, Carolina
AG:	Angel González, Mayagüez
BR:	Bárbara Rodríguez, central Puerto Rico
BS:	Brígida Sotomayor Vargas, Mayagüez
BV:	Brunilda Vargas Muñiz, Mayagüez
CC:	Carmen Colón de Jorge, Luquillo
CM:	Cruz María Santiago, Morovis
CMM:	Carmen María Morales Serrano, Orocovis
CR:	Cheo Rodríguez, central Puerto Rico
CV:	Carmen Vega, Mayagüez
CVS:	Camila Vargas viuda de Sotomayor, Mayagüez
DB:	Doña Bolina (Rafaela Parrilla), Loíza Aldea
DC:	Doña Casimira (Casimira Osoris Fuentes), Loíza Aldea
FB:	Félix Nicholás Beato, Fajardo
GS:	Eugenio Santiago Marrero, Morovis
IL:	Irenio López Mercado, Las Marías
IV:	Inés Vargas Muñiz, Mayagüez
JP:	Josefina Pizarro, Carolina
JS:	Julia Santiago, Carolina
LF:	Luisa Flores Rivera, Mayagüez
MC:	María Cruz Avilés, Orocovis
ML:	María Lagoa de González, Mayagüez
MO:	María Otero Collazo viuda de Santiago, Morovis
MOS:	Ramona Ortíz Santana, Carolina
MS:	María Salgado, Carolina
MSM:	Mercedes Sotomayor viuda de Martell, Mayagüez
PA:	Petra Angleró, Mayagüez
PC:	Pepe Chávez, Rio Piedras Estación Experimental (botanical gardens)
PN:	Francisco (Panky) Negrón Maldonado, Caguas
PR:	Providencia Rivera Rodríguez, Loíza Aldea
PS:	Primi Socorro Vargas, Mayagüez
PV:	Paula Valentín Mercado, Las Marías
TR:	Tato Rodríguez Valentín, Las Marías

Healing Lore and More at a Glance

Alcohol & Drug Addiction

CR&BR: Every time you have the urge to drink alcohol, drink a glass of lemon juice.

AND Eat as much raw garlic as you can to counteract the poisonous effects of alcohol and other drugs.

AND When withdrawing from an addiction to alcohol or other drugs, drink calming teas (*guarapos*) like those made from the leaves of the sour orange tree (*naranjo*).

AND Calcium-rich foods are calming, as they support the nervous system. Try seaweed, cooked nettle leaves, sesame!

MC: Catch a dozen *fliches*, those insects that scoot around on the top of the water. Toast them a bit in a pot so that they get reddish, and leave them for eight days in a bottle of rum. (The rum will turn pink.) Then strain the contents of that bottle into an empty one and make a gift of that "special" bottle to the person with the drinking problem. That person will get a tremendous case of diarrhea and nausea, but s/he may thank you for it because s/he'll never touch rum again.

Allergies

DB: Drink lots of cooling teas, such as *paletaria*, purslane (*verdolaga*), amaranth (*blero*), black nightshade (*mata gallina*), and spineless (*tuna*) cactus.

Animal Bites & Stings

BV: Crush some garlic (*ajo*) and put it on the bite so it won't swell up.

PS&M: When stung by wasps or jellyfish, apply fresh urine "straight" or mixed with clay-ish earth to make a poultice. Commercial ammonia is also good.

M: Make a simple poultice of common plantain (*llantén*) by chewing up a couple of leaves and placing them on bites, stings or cuts. If the problem is on a small area of the body, like a finger or toe, you can use a whole plantain leaf to tie the little poultice on.

Arthritis & Rheumatism

AG: Drink the juice of a lemon mixed with water every day, once or twice a day.

PC: Add arnica flowers, camphor (*alcanfor*) leaves or pastilles, bay rum (*malagueta*) and eucalyptus (*eucalipto*) leaves to *alcoholado* and massage the ailing joints.

MSM: Boil the new leaves and woody stems of the native lentil (*gandul*) bush and take as tea, two cups a day for two weeks.

MO: Boil up some grated ginger in cooking oil and rub into arthritic joints.

ML: Mash the yellow flowers of the *roble amarillo* and massage them into the painful area *OR* make a poultice of the mashed flowers, wrapping them close to the painful area.

OR Make a liniment by filling a jar with rosemary (*romero*), *poleo* and marjoram (*mejorana*), and then covering it with *amoniaco* (an ammoniated solution used for rubdowns) plus a little *Aguarrás* (a petroleum distillate used for rubs). Let steep for two or three weeks, and use it to massage painful back muscles.

PA: Add bay rum leaves (*malagueta*) and camphor (*alcanfor*)—leaves or crushed pastilles—to *alcoholado* and let it sit a few weeks. Use as a massage liniment.

ML: Rub lemon juice or almond oil over the painful joints.

PV: Rub the grease of a guinea hen into the joints as if it were lotion.

IL: For rheumatic pains, add *pata de perro*, a type of *cadillo* or bur, to a therapeutic bath. (See **Baths** for instructions.)

GS: Add basil (*albahaca*) to *alcoholado*, let sit a week or so, and give yourself cooling rubs.

OR Take a therapeutic bath! (See **Baths** for instructions.)

Asthma & Lung Congestion

PA: Mash up the stems of elder (*saúco*) to extract the juice. For every two tablespoons of that juice, mix a teaspoon of cooking oil and a pinch of salt. Take it several times a day.

OR Put a litre of aloe gel (from about five or six large, fleshy leaves) into a glass or ceramic bowl. Add a cup of honey and a cup of spices such as star anise, whole cloves and cinammon. Add a cup of rum to preserve it, and keep refrigerated. In ten days or two weeks it is ready to take, a tablespoon or two at a time. Besides asthma, it's also good for indigestion.

IV: Boil three *poleo* leaves, one peeled and chopped "leaf" of aloe vera (*sábila*), and a pinch of anise seeds (*anís*) in two cups of water for ten or fifteen minutes on a low flame. Prepare and drink as needed.

MO: Boil up two succulent *malá* leaves with a few anise stars in a cup and a half of water for about fifteen minutes, and then drink it. That will get rid of phlegm and blood too.

OR For a desperate cough, even whooping cough, boil up snake plant (*chucho*) root in water or in coconut water and take it as needed.

OR Add a little witch hazel solution (*Agua Maravilla*) to any remedy to help eliminate phlegm from the lungs.

OR Drink *ipecacuana* tea: three small pieces of leaf to a cup and a half of water for about ten minutes. Will cause you to vomit up the phlegm in your chest.

OR Take a tablespoon of cooking oil every morning, and the problem is eliminated litle by little.

OR First rub the chest with a cloth soaked in *alcoholado*. Then put plenty of *numoticina* (a rubefacient used in chest plasters) on top of that cloth with some camphorated oil (*aceite alcanforado*). Cover that poultice well, with cotton and then a shirt. Let the person sweat and sweat.

OR For even the most serious bronchial complaint: Mix a 4 oz. bottle of each of the seven syrups (*los siete jarabes*) including *ipecacuana* syrup, chicory (*achicoria*) syrup, cocillana syrup (*jarabe pectoral*), balsam (*tolú*) syrup, star anise (*anís de estrella*), anise seed (*anís de grano*) and witch hazel solution (*Agua Maravilla*). Then add the gelatin of three fat aloe vera (*sábila*) leaves. Add a cup of the juice of both watercress (*berro*) and *poleo*, then add some almond or cooking oil and some honey. Finally, add a little rum or anisette in order to preserve it. When you're done, you should have a gallon of liquid. Let it sit in the refrigerator for five or six days, then drink the gallon over a week's time.

PV&PR: Peel and chop up a leaf of aloe vera (*sábila*) and put it in a small jug of water. Leave it outside during the night, and drink that water during the day. You may add lemon and honey to the drink.

IV: Boil the papery covering and ends of two whole garlic (*ajo*) heads with two shoots of *poleo* and a small handful of linden (*tilo*) flowers. Take with honey to taste.

GS: Rub tallow (*sebo Flandes*) into a porous piece of cloth and apply the cloth to the person's chest, or put the *sebo Flandes* directly onto the skin and then cover it up with cloth.

OR Try strong teas of *poleo*.

BV: Add either the juice of aloe vera (*sábila*) or common plantain (*llantén*) leaves to herbal teas to get rid of lung congestion.

OR For a more serious complaint, take a small handful of *cohitre blanco*, a chopped up "leaf" of spineless (*tuna*) cactus, some red mint leaves (*yerba buena*) and chamomile (*manzanilla*) flowers, some chopped up ginger (*jengibre dulce*), a small handful of *poleo* leaves, a small handful of *paletaria*, two juicy aloe vera (*sábila*) leaves, and a small handful of white basil (*albahaca blanca*). Wash everything and cook it up all together, covered, for about twenty minutes in half a gallon of water. Add two tablespoons of witch hazel solution (*Agua Maravilla*) and take with honey as needed.

OR Drink teas of wild zinnia (*escopetón*).

CC: Make a vapor bath by boiling eucalyptus (*eucalipto*) and rosemary (*romero*) for fifteen minutes in a pot on the stove. Turn off the flame, and breathe in the steam from the pot as deeply as you can. Cover your head with a towel so that no steam escapes.

JP: Peel some thick aloe (*sábila*) leaves. Cut the inside gelatin up in pieces, put it in a bowl with a little witch hazel solution and some honey, and let it sit a few days so that the plant's medicinal qualities are dissolved in the liquid. Take tablespoons of it as needed to loosen the phlegm from your chest.

PV: Boil early green leaves of *ipecacuana* with red mint (*yerba buena*) or lemon balm (*toronjil*) or marjoram (*mejorana*). Take as tea. It really gets rid of phlegm.

IV: If a person has trouble breathing, warm two large or five small leaves of the life plant (*bruja*) over a flame or rising steam. Then squeeze the juice into a small saucepan with two cups water and boil for 15 minutes. Add a pinch of salt before serving.

AC: For a bad cough, drink papaya flower tea with honey.

PC: To alleviate asthma, boil Puerto Rico's national flower, *flor de maga* as a tea, and drink throughout the day.

AND For a bad cough, boil up the flower of the shell plant (*pimienta Angola*) with some mint leaves and drink as needed.

Baths
for bodily aches, fever, spiritual cleansing and renewal, relaxation, good luck, and more

GS: For a bath to treat body pain and illness, fill a big vat with water, and put in all the plants once the water boils. You might include eucalyptus (*eucalipto*) and sour orange leaves (*el naranjo*), *santa María*, mugwort (*altamisa*) and many more. You have to be clean already before taking the bath, and you can't just throw the water every which place, either. You have to start at the top, at the head, and cover the entire body. That's how you receive the water. Afterwards, you don't wash with soap, ever.

PV&TR: For a bath to treat fever, body pains, and other physical and mental complaints, first you find the leaves and roots you want to use: Caribbean vervain (*verbena*), palma Christi (*higuereta*), bitter ginger (*jengibre amargo*), *higuillo oloroso*, *rompecota*, a little bit of everything. Use about three little handfuls of plant material for five gallons of water, and boil the plants for a good half hour. Then, when that liquid is no longer too hot, strain it, then go into the shower and have someone pour that bath over your entire body in a running stream of cleansing water. After the bath, you can't rinse yourself off or anything, because you don't want to dilute the benefits of the plants.

MO: Pick roses and all the other flowers that are around, along with the leaves of avocado (*aguacate*), mango (*mangó*), coffee (*café*), *higuillo oloroso*, and more. Boil them all up in a pot as if you were making a big soup, then leave it for the next day, or at least a few hours so that it's not too hot. After you've taken a bath for cleanliness, get into the tub and receive the stream of water as it is poured down over you from your head to your feet.

BV: First the person gets all soaped up. (The strained bath water you prepare will be used to rinse the soap off your entire body.) After letting the bath water run over his or her entire body, wrap the person up in warm clothes and blankets to encourage heavy sweating. The very process of sweating helps to eliminate the illness.

For muscle aches, use baths of mugwort (*altamisa*), *higuillo oloroso, vara prieta, campana, tártago*, and bay rum (*malagueta*).

PS&BV: Use *vara prieta* along with *cariaquillo* and mango leaves to make a bath to remove all negative energies. It's also good for muscle aches and rheumatism.

DC: First you have to boil the plants you'll be using, and let that water cool. Then after bathing yourself with soap and water, you let the plant bath flow over you from your head to your toes, over every part of your body. Get out of the tub without drying yourself off. You can't sit in the water, because the water has taken with it all the negativity that you don't want or need any longer.

For luck, bathe in white basil (*albahaca*), red mint (*yerba buena*) and marjoram (*mejorana*).

To counteract or offset spiritual problems or even manipulation by others, use *poleo*, wormseed (*pazote*), *salvia*, mugwort (*altamisa*), aloe (*sábila*), and Caribbean vervain (*verbena*).

ML: Use sour orange leaves (*naranjo*), albahaca (*basil*), *salvia*, *curía*, marjoram (*mejorana*), red mint (*yerba buena*) and rosemary (*romero*) as a healing, aromatic bath.

DB: If you think you have something like bad energy following you around, take a bath of marjoram (*mejorana*), Florida water (*Agua de Florida*), red mint (*yerba buena*) or mugwort (*altamisa*).

OR Swim in the ocean to cleanse the body and soul of all negativity.

For relaxation, bathe with special, soothing herbs like mugwort (*altamisa*) and sour orange leaves (*hojas de naranjo*).

JS: To make an unboiled bath for a child with fever, squeeze the juice of fresh aloe vera (*sábila*), *poleo*, mugwort (*altamisa*), garlic weed (*anamú*) and other plants into a five gallon bucket of water. Add some alcohol to the water and put it outside in a strong sun. Within half an hour or so it's ready for a bath. If there are no camphor (*alcanfor*) leaves around, you can add half a camphor pastille to the water and that makes it even fresher. After having been bathed with the stream of fragrant water, the child gets wrapped so that he can sweat as much as possible.

CR: Choose plants according to knowledge and intuition. Go out of doors to collect plants for a bath, and notice, "the *santa María* is in flower; I must take some for my bath," or "over there the *cariaquillo* seems to be beckoning." Prepare your bath according to what is happening in the moment. Boil, for 15 or 20 minutes, the leaves, stems, flowers and roots you've chosen, and add them to the person's bath water. Sprinkle some fresh flowers on top. Have the person listen to soothing music while bathing. Let the person feel completely safe and taken care of. Then see what happens.

Blood Stains

MO: Pour a bottle of witch hazel solution (*Agua Maravilla*) in with your clothes as you wash them, and the blood comes right out.

Boils & External Cysts

CM: Using some light paper or a feather, paint the boil or tumor with the yolk of an egg. Put some towels underneath the area to absorb the liquid when the boil opens.

MO: Heat a leaf or more of garlic weed (*el anamú*) and use it as a hot compress for a growth that won't burst open.

GS: Almost any leaf heated up can be used to break open a boil or tumorous growth, because it's the heat, actually, that does the work. You can use hot leaves or hot cloths, even a hot, cooked egg. And as the growth opens up with the heat, you feel a tremendous relief.

PS: Boil up some *tuatúa* leaves for about 15 minutes. While that water is cooling, warm and soften up a large, fresh leaf by passing it back and forth over a low flame. Wash the area with the warm "tea," then put the warm leaf on the cyst. You may want to cover it with a little oil in order to keep it stuck to the skin, and/or you may want to use a towel to hold the leaf on. The leaf will draw whatever is causing the problem inside, out to the surface. After the boil explodes, wash the area with more warm *tuatúa* water and apply an antiseptic cream.

OR Follow the same procedure using mallow leaves (*malva*). You can also drink the mallow water.

ML: Wrap the warm, mashed pulp of the tuberose (*azucena*) root onto the area with a cloth.

Broken Bones & Sprains

PA: For sprains, heat up the leaves of Madeira vine (*sueldaconsuelda*) with the steam from your teapot. Then chop them up and mix them in a little bowl with warm cooking oil. Apply that poultice all over the affected area, and cover it with gauze or other fabric. Leave on for two days before changing. If a bone is broken, and there is no cast, apply the Madeira vine poultice after the bone has been set.

LF: Grate the yam-like roots of *sueldaconsuelda,* and add some milky liquid from the breadfruit (*pana*) and some olive or almond oil. Once the bone has been set, this is used as a poultice, tied on with cotton or silk fabric to keep it in place. It is said to help the bones "knit" together.

Bruises, Bumps

PS: Wrap the bruised area with rags soaked in cold salt water.

OR If the skin swells and blackens without going down after two or three days, use rags soaked with very hot salt water to bring down the swelling.

MO: Chop or mash up the leaves of the oyster plant (*sanguinaria*) and mix that up with some salt. Then apply it to the bruise as a poultice.

OR Apply the ashes of the large and leafy *bálsamo* tree.

JS: Mix butter, sugar and salt in proportions of 2:2:1. Apply that mixture to the wound, and there will be no swelling.

Burns

JS: Grate raw potato and use as a poultice on the burned area. It's very cooling. If you apply the poultice directly after burning yourself, the burn won't blister, and you might not even lose any hair from the burned spot.

BS: Rub the juice of aloe vera (*sábila*) all over the burned skin, frequently.

Callouses & Corns

PS: Rub the sap of *tártago* on corns or callouses with a little piece of cotton, daily.

ML: Wrap the mashed pulp of the tuberose (*azucena*) root around the corns with a cloth.

Calming the Nerves

BR: Eat calcium-rich foods, such as seaweed, nettle leaves, sesame; there are many sources besides milk!

PV: Drink chamomile (*manzanilla*) or sour orange leaf (*naranjo*) teas.

DB: Drink special soothing teas of linden tree flowers (*tilo*), chamomile (*manzanilla*) or sour orange tree leaves (*naranjo*).

PS: Take teas of valerian (*valeriana*) root.

Cancer
(at the onset and/or for relief of pain)

DC: Drink the boiled seeds of *cundeamor* with shoots of garlic weed (*anamú*) and leaves of common plantain (*llantén*).

BV: Extract the juice of a handful of *anamú* leaves and another handful of common plantain (*llantén*) by adding both to a blender along with a cup and a half of water. Strain and take twice daily.

Chewing Gum

BV: Make a cut in a breadfruit (*pana*) tree. The next day, you'll have some sap to chew as natural gum.

Childbirth

during labor

BV: Drink nutmeg (*nemocá*) tea and apply wraps of cloth soaked in analgesic ointments like "belladona" and *triaca* "ointment of the air" for the pain.

MC: Take a strong tea of anise (*anís*) seeds with the flowers and leaves of coffee senna (*hedionda chiquita*). It will help to eliminate gas, and if there's pain, the tea will relieve the pain as well.

post-partum tonics & care

PA. The calabash (*higüera*) or white gourd medicine is actually a type of tisane. The traditional way of making it is this: First, bore a hole in one end of a large, unripe, white calabash and pour into that hole as many whole cloves (*clavo de especia*), anise seeds (*anís de grano*) and anise stars (*anís de estrella*) as fit into one's hand. Then, bury the gourd for a couple of days until a liquid forms inside. That's part of the medicine. The spices keep the gourd from going bad, but it does ferment a little. If you want to be more modern, you can make it by scooping the flesh and seeds from the gourd, putting it all in a glass bowl, adding the spices and leaving it in the refrigerator for a few days before offering it to the woman.

Any way it's prepared, she should take it (liquid and solid) for about nine days straight, about a cup a day, and during that time she should really rest. In fact, if she wants to preserve her womb, she shouldn't do any heavy work at all for a full 40 days!

AC: Boil up half a bar of bittersweet chocolate with two cups of water and eight or ten leaves of red mint (*yerba buena*) for about 15 minutes. Drink to help strengthen the womb after birth.

MO: When a woman gives birth and part of the placenta remains inside, a sitz bath of boiled palma Christi (*higuereta*) leaves will help to clean her out.

IL: After childbirth, a vaginal wash of boiled mallow (*malva*) leaves with a few drops of almond oil gently soothes and cleanses.

BV: After the birth, drink lots of chicken broth with burnt bread.

Circulation

PS: To improve the circulation, take ginger (*jengibre dulce*) tea.

M: Exercise.

BV: Boil up the leaves of annato (*achiote*) and soak legs and feet for poor circulation or muscle spasms.

Clear Mind

DB: Take teas made of the leaves and (unsprayed) skin of the *jobo* fruit.

AND Relax.

Coagulate Milk

BV: To coagulate milk quickly for making cheese, add the little fruits of the *maya* plant or lemon juice to the milk.

Coffee Substitute

GS: Toast the seeds of coffee senna (*hedionda*) over a low flame so they don't burn. Then grind them and boil them up. Delicious!

Colds

CM: Rub chest with some warm Vicks and drink eucalyptus (*eucalipto*) or ginger (*jengibre dulce*) tea mixed with warming spices such as cloves (*clavo de especia*) and cinammon (*canela*).

AC: At the onset of a cold, drink hot lemon juice with a half teaspoon of witch hazel solution (*Agua Maravilla*).

MO: Take teas of yellow elder (*saúco amarillo*) stems and flowers.

OR Teas of *anacagüita* flowers.

OR Teas of *cariaquillo*.

OR Boil some chopped ginger in just a little water for ten minutes or so, and add to hot milk. Season with honey.

PV: Take tea of elder flowers (*saúco*) with orange leaves and ginger (*jengibre dulce*). Add honey, if you like.

OR Strong teas of *poleo*.

GS: Teas of wild jessamine (*yapaná*) get rid of any coldness in the body, and related conditions.

DB: Drink star anise (*anís de estrella*) tea with honey and lemon.

OR To get rid of a condition of cold in the body, wrap dry coffee mixed with cooking oil around the forehead with a towel.

BV: Take teas of sour orange leaves (*naranjo*).

ML: For a "watery" cold with runny eyes and nose, mix lemon juice, honey and rum in equal parts. Heat and take as needed.

Colic

IV: Make a tea of cabbage leaves (three leaves in three cups of water, boiled 15 minutes) and half a teaspoon of anise (*anís*) seeds.

PA: Give the baby a tea of cabbage leaves with a pinch of salt.

DB: Warm up a leaf of the castor bean plant (*higuereta*), rub cooking oil on it, and place on the child's belly, covered with a towel.

CVS: Give the child a weak tea of *tártago* leaf buds.

Complexion

AC: Let raw rice sit in a little bit of water until it softens, then mash up until it forms a paste. Use paste as facial mask.

PS: Rub aloe vera (*sábila*) juice on spots and blemishes.
OR To moisturize a dry complexion, massage avocado into the skin and leave as a mask for twenty minutes to half an hour before rinsing well.
OR Rub lemon on oily skin to cut grease and eliminate dark spots.

Constipation

JP: Drink teas made from the young leaf buds of *tártago*.

JS: For children, first give the child a teaspoon of cooking oil. Then rub the little hairs off a few stems of *cohitre blanco*, press the stems into a ball shape, cover with cooking oil, and use as a suppository.

DB: Drink lots of coconut water with lemon.

ML: Eat tamarind (*tamarindo*) fruits raw or drink the syrupy juice made by soaking them in water and then blending them with that water in liquifier.
OR Break up a pod of purging cassia (*caña fístula*) and boil up a small piece, a few inches long in a cup or two of water. Take in very small amounts.

IL: Make a "towel poultice" of mallow leaves (*malva*). Simply boil the leaves as if for a *guarapo*, then soak a towel in that warm solution, wring it out, and let it rest upon the abdomen.

MOS: Mix the sap of a leaf of aloe vera (*sábila*) with a washed and chopped leaf of spineless (*tuna*) cactus in the blender with two cups of water. Add honey and drink throughout the day.

AND Eat fresh, fibrous foods, nothing canned.

AND Eat your last meal by 6 PM so that your food has a chance to fully digest and doesn't ferment as you sleep.

M: Take a puff or two of a freshly dried, homemade cigar.

Cooling, Nourishing Drinks (will increase urination)

MS: Peel and cut up a fat leaf of the spineless (*tuna*) cactus and then put the pieces in water in a jar in the refrigerator. Instead of drinking water from the faucet, drink the cactus water.

OR Pick and wash a handful of *prenetaria*, put it in a jar of water in the fridge, and drink instead of tap water.

GS: Drink teas of *paletaria*, *cojitre blanco* and purslane (*verdolaga*) either separately or mixed in any combination.

BV: For a condition of inner heat or inflammation, cook up one big "leaf" of the spineless (*tuna*) cactus with a handful of coarse, raw corn in a litre of water and then drink it, as if it were regular drinking water or juice.

CM: Rinse mallow (*malva*) leaves and put them in a pitcher of water. Leave in the refrigerator and drink as desired throughout the day.

Cuts, Wounds & Sores

CM: Wash with warm salt water. Should be the saltiness of half a cup of water with one or two teaspoonfuls of salt. Good for animal bites, bad cuts, etc.

TR: Bathe the open sore, cut or wound with a "tea" of *guaco*. It kills germs.

JS: After you've washed the wound well, sprinkle it with the dried and pulverized leaf of *yerba cangá*.

PS: For bloody wounds, apply wood ashes mixed with dry, well ground and roasted coffee, wrapped up in rags.

BV: For a cut, chop up a leaf of *sueldaconsuelda*, mix it with cooking oil, and stick it to the wound as a poultice.

OR Mash up the thick leaves of malá and tie them on to the cut to stop the bleeding. Then for rapid curing, apply Humphrey's Udder Balm, belladona ointment or kerosene that's been burned for three or four hours in a lantern. Kerosene is especially good for animals because besides speeding up the healing process, it keeps flies out of their wounds.

LF: For suppurating sores on the legs, extract the juice of wild eggplant leaves in a blender with a bit of water, strain the liquid, soak a towel in that liquid, and use the towel as a poultice.

Diabetes
(to lower blood sugar)

JS: Boil up five mulberry (*morera*) leaves for fifteen minutes in about three cups of water, and drink it every day.

MO&GS: Drink teas of the leaves and stems of native lentils (*gandules*).

OR Make a tea of sweet verbena (*yerba dulce*) root with *cundeamor*, then put it in the refrigerator and drink it all day long.

BV: Drink *guarapos* of native lentil (*gandul*) buds or almond leaves as if they were water, cold during the day, warmed up at night.

ML: Drink teas of broadleaf coriander (*culantro del monte*).

OR Drink teas of the leaf buds of the tropical almond (*almendra*) and *caimito* trees.

CC: Make a green juice by mixing (in the blender) about three handfuls of the following greens: *cundeamor*, native lentil (*gandul*) leaves, stinging nettle (*ortiga brava*)—wear gloves when picking nettles—and lemon grass (*limoncillo*) with three cups of water. Strain and drink three times a day.

Diarrhea

CM: Drink a strong, green tea of black nightshade (*mata gallina*) with *sal de heno* (a sodium bicarbonate-based digestive).

JP: Put raw rice in water and leave it there for an hour or more. Drink the rice water.

DC: Take teas of white basil (*albahaca blanca*) mixed with cashew (*pajuil*) husks and *hicaco* fruit.

BV: Take teas of Caribbean vervain (*verbena*) with lemon.

LF: Sip teas of the small, new leaves of *tártago* mixed with oregano (*oregano chiquito*).

Digestive Aids
(hints for good digestion)

GS: You can eat all you want, but you should wait until it's time to eat. Because if you have a big lunch at noon and you eat again at 1:30, you're interfering with the process of digestion. And that's the cause of lots of troubles.

MO: Eat slowly.

IV: Take the juice of a lemon in water twice daily if you have trouble digesting greasy foods.

PS: Eat lemon along with heavy, greasy foods like shellfish.

Dying

CMM: When a dying person is in pain, chop up a couple of handfuls of red mint (*yerba buena*) and boil for fifteen minutes or so in enough milk to cover the herb. Soak a cloth in that milk while it's still warm and apply it to the person's stomach. This smells good, comforts, strengthens, and helps to reduce pain.

Earache

AC: Warm a leaf of the life plant (*bruja*) and squeeze the warm juice into your ear. Cover it up with some cotton if desired.

BV: Warm up a leaf of *bruja*, then crush it and soak up the juice with a little piece of cotton. Put the piece of cotton in your ear while it's still warm. As the liquid from the cotton seeps out into the ear, the pain goes away.

MO&ML: Warm up some marjoram (*mejorana*) leaves and chop them up. Pick up their warm juice with a pad of cotton and squeeze it into the ear. Cover it up with the cotton.

Edema

MOS: When someone has swollen legs and ankles, boil the stems and leaves of the tamarind (*tamarindo*) tree, and when the water is warm to hot, soak the legs in that water, up to the knees.

OR Drink the water as tea.

CMM: Drink teas of new soursop (*guanábana*) leaves.

Erysipelas

CM: Pick the leaves of stinging vine (*pringamosa*) with gloves, then cook them up in some oil in a frying pan on a very low flame for five or ten minutes or until the oil turns green. Then use a feather or something similar to paint that oil all over the irritated skin.

Eyes

MO: For clouded vision, place a few of basil's (*albahaca*) tiny seeds in the inside corners of the eyes, very gently, so that they don't irritate. Leave them a while so that they can attract mucus and foreign matter.

DB: For cloudy vision, put some well-rinsed leaves of common plantain (*llantén*) alone or with rue (*ruda*) in a clean glass of water, and leave outside or on your window ledge during the cool dampness of the night. When you get up in the morning, wash your eyes with that water.

BV: For conjunctivitis, leave half a dozen fairy roses (*rosa cienhojas*) in a small cup of water overnight, and rinse the eyes with that water throughout the day.

PA: Cool purslane (*verdolaga*) tea makes an excellent eye wash.

Fatigue & Weakness

IV: Before cooking a chicken for soup (should be a free-range, native chicken), cut it up and cut the bones too, so that the marrow can be cooked right into the broth. You can prepare the broth with the meat too if you want, or cook the meat aside. The marrow is the most important part of the soup! Strain and drink.

JS: Drink dove or pigeon broth every day for two or three weeks.

DB: Drink daily punches made from a couple of fresh, raw eggs, a cup of fresh milk, half an ounce of brandy or rum, and some brown sugar.

Fertilizer

PN: Use alluvial soil and cured manure. Chicken manure must cure for over a year before it can be used.

MO: Add coffee grounds and potato peelings to manure as it's curing.

Fever
(also see Baths)

MO: Take teas of *gran señora*.

OR Teas of lemon grass (*limoncillo*).

OR Teas of Caribbean vervain (*verbena*).

OR Take two pieces of tissue (the wrapping kind) paper just a little bigger than the soles of the person's feet. Rub beef tallow (*sebo Flandes*) into the paper. Then take a little salt, a little sugar, and roll a bottle over it until it's ground up fine. Put the powdered salt and sugar on top of the paper covered with tallow and sprinkle some cooking oil on top of all that. Next, you prepare a bandage (to be tied onto the person's forehead) exactly the same way. Then you light a candle and use it to warm the bandage (don't put it too close, of course), and put the bandage on the person's head. Do the same with the papers, and put them on the soles of the person's feet. Finally, you put on some warm socks, and the person goes to sleep. The person should sleep as much as s/he wants, and don't take off those little paper soles until the next day. That's the remedy for stubborn fevers that simply won't go down. It always works!

PV: Take teas of Caribbean vervain (*verbena*) and common plantain (*llantén*).

OR Peel and mash up lemon grass root (*limoncillo*), and then boil it up with *anís*. Drink as needed.

OR Drink teas of the leaves of sour orange (*naranjo*) with *poleo* and yellow elder (*saúco amarillo*).

OR Stick *salvia* leaves on to the soles of your feet, with camphor cream (*alcanfor*) and stick another leaf on your forehead. Lie down covered by a blanket. Also works for headaches.

OR Take teas of black nightshade (*mata gallina*) mixed with Caribbean vervain (*la verbena*).

PS: Take teas of *gran señora* alone or with *botón de cadete*.

BV: Common plantain (*llantén*) and *curía* cut fever and pain. Can be added to any tea.

OR Take teas of chamomile (*manzanilla*) with red mint (*yerba buena*) and black nightshade (*mata gallina*). To that decoction add some well washed and chopped-up *tuna* cactus, which is cooling. Drink all day long, as if it were water.

CVS: Run a little "bath" of the fresh urine of a young child over the forehead of the person who has the fever, and then rub the forehead with tallow (*sebo de Flandes*).

DC: Administer the juice of the chicory plant (*achicoria*) by the tablespoonful.

OR Offer chicory tea (entire plant).

PC: Take teas of *quinino del pobre*.

Flu

MC: Drink fragrant geranium (*geranio oloroso*) tea.

GS: Drink strong teas of *poleo*.

BV: Take *guarapos* of *gran señora* or *botón de cadete* mixed with lemon grass (*limoncillo*), which improves flavor while it cuts fever.

OR For a flu with a cough, take a handful of *cohitre blanco*, a chopped up "leaf" of spineless (*tuna*) cactus, some red mint leaves (*yerba buena*) and chamomile (*manzanilla*) flowers, a small handful of *paletaria*, two juicy aloe vera (*sábila*) leaves, and a handful of white basil (*albahaca blanca*). Wash everything and cook it up all together, covered, for about twenty minutes in two litres of water. Take with honey as needed.

PA: For flu, take teas of the root and leaf of lemon grass (*limoncillo*).

OR Mulberry leaf (*morera*) tea.

ML: Chop up sour orange (*naranjo*) fruit and the white, inside part of the rind, and add to any "flu formula" leafy, green tea. This will help to bring down the fever.

OR Grate a green papaya and boil it for five to ten minutes, covered, over a low flame. Drink the juice.

OR Take teas of eucalyptus (*eucalipto*) leaves.

OR For a flu with cough, take teas of *curía*.

OR Prepare a large *menorativa* for the whole family with the root of Puerto Rican royal palm (*palma real*), coconut palm (*palma de coco*), a carrot, a small, green papaya, a small piece of purging cassia (*cañafístula*), and—from the pharmacy—*maná canelón* (a sweet, cinammony flavoring agent used often in children's medicine). Everyone takes a cup. That cleans out the system and helps to prevent and/or get rid of the flu.

Fowls' "Pip"

AC&JS: Add orange rind or lemon juice to birds' water supply.

Full Harvest

PN: Always plant during the waning moon (only sugar cane and yucca can be planted at any time of month).

AND Take seeds from banana trees during low tide (to be planted during the waning moon).

Hair

AC: To help hair grow: boil up some Caribbean vervain (*verbena*), let it cool off, and use this "tea" as a final hair rinse after shampoo. Leave it in until next shampoo and repeat.

JP&PA: Rosemary (*romero*) boiled up and applied after shampoo as a final rinse adds body and gives your hair a nice dark color. It also prevents hair from falling out.

AC: To give hair body, and to get rid of dandruff: peel a large stalk of aloe vera (*sábila*), cut it up into tiny pieces, add to three or four cups of water and leave it all in the refrigerator. The next day, beat the mixture, strain it, apply it to the hair after shampooing, and don't rinse it out. You can make a lot and store in the refrigerator for future rinses.

BR: For dandruff, collect stinging nettle (*ortiga brava*) with gloves so as not to get stung. Then crush the leaves in a mortar and pestle or using a rolling pin. Place crushed leaves and juice in water, and let sit for three or four hours. Later, strain the water, pour it over the scalp after shampooing, and leave it there without rinsing it off. If you make a lot, it will keep in the refrigerator.

AND For baldness, massage daily with a rosemary (*romero*) oil made this way. Fill a jar with fresh, organic rosemary. Then cover it with olive oil and let it sit for six weeks. Regular, brisk massages with that oil will stimulate hair growth.

BV: For dandruff, use the raw juice of aloe vera (*sábila*) as if it were shampoo.

PS: When someone starts losing hair, massage scalp regularly with coconut oil.

PS: For head lice, boil up some vines of *cundeamor* until the water turns dark green; then use it as if it were a shampoo, but leave it on the person's head for a good 15 or 20 minutes. That kills the lice, and it's good for the scalp.

Headaches

JS: Grate some raw potato and mix it up with some witch hazel solution (*Agua Maravilla*) to make a cooling paste. Put it on your forehead, temples and neck, and lie down for a little while. What relief!

GS: For a headache caused by heat that needs to be drawn out, rub a leaf of annato (*achiote*) with cooking oil and stick it on to your forehead. If it's working, the leaf will dry out and break up until it's powder. If it stays wet and slides around, it's not the remedy you need.

PS: For a migraine, heat up some *salvia* leaves, enough to cover the entire forehead and temples. Then add a paste of roasted coffee and cooking oil on top of the leaves, and tie it all on with a towel. Lie down for a few hours with that bandage tied onto your head.

IL: Place *salvia* leaves coated with camphorated oil or ointment, Vicks, or cooking oil on the forehead and temples. Lie down.

MO: For migraine headache, put a mixture of native wood ashes and salt in a bucket of hot water. Wrap the person's forehead in a bandage soaked in that mixture, and put his legs, from the knees down, into the bucket. Both the water on his legs and the bandage on his forehead must be really hot.

PV: Place your feet in a big bucket of hot water.

IL: Place *salvia* leaves on the forehead, neck and temples. You can use cooking oil, camphorated oil or Vicks to make them stick and increase the effect.

Heart

GS: After a heart attack, place a warmed-up leaf of *corazón* over the heart. The same leaf, taken in the form of medicinal teas, will also prevent further attacks.

Hemorrhage

MO: Take *guarapos* of common plantain (*llantén*).

BV: Drink teas of *malá* or chew the leaves.

High Blood Pressure

JS: Every day, in a litre of water, boil up five leaves of spiny cilantro (*recao*) with the outer peel and ends of three heads of garlic, plus five common plantain leaves and five sour orange leaves for fifteen minutes or until the flavor is strong. Then, instead of drinking tap water, drink that herb water, cold if you like, from the fridge.

MO: Drink broadleaf coriander (*culantro del monte*) tea daily.

PS: Cut a *jagua* fruit in quarters, put it in a pitcher of water in the refrigerator and, after a day or so, drink the water. No sugar needed! Keep a large supply on hand.

B&CR: Eat raw garlic daily.

PV: Eat parcha and drink the juice.

CVS: Drink teas of the young leaves of the guava bush (*guayabo*).

Indigestion

MS: Take a tea of *guanábana* leaves with *poleo*.

AC: Drink a tea of new mango leaves mixed with *guanábana* leaves.

PV: Try a tea of chamomile flowers (*manzanilla*).
OR Teas of lemon balm (*toronjil*) and red mint (*yerba buena*) combined for nausea. If there's no lemon balm or red mint around, try a tea of sour orange leaves (*hoja de naranjo*).

MOS: Put a pinch of wood ash in a cup of water. Let the ashes settle for a while, then drink that water with half a teaspoonful of cooking oil.

CM: Drink a strong, green tea of black nightshade (*mata gallina*) with *tuatúa*.

GS: Take teas of red mint (*yerba buena*). They're good and cooling for the stomach.

MO: Take anise (*anís*) seed teas.
OR Teas of Caribbean vervain (*verbena*) root.
OR Teas of lemon balm (*toronjil*).

GS: If you want to throw up, drink a tea made of three *tártago* leaves which you've picked by pulling upward from the stems. To settle your stomach, make the same tea but take the leaves by pulling them downward.

DC: Drink mint (*menta*) tea.
OR Teas of red mint (*yerba buena*), *poleo* and *guanábana* buds.

BV: Take teas of red mint (*yerba buena*), chamomile (*manzanilla*) and *paletaria*, alone, or in combination.
OR Caribbean vervain (*verbena*) tea with lemon.

ML: If you feel as though food is rotting in your stomach, drink cooling coconut water.

CMM: Take teas of *corazón* leaves, either alone or with the leaf buds of the guava bush (*guayabo*) and sour orange (*naranjo*) tree leaves. This will help for gas as well as indigestion and nausea.
OR Poleo tea.

Infertility (women)

BV: For a "condition of congested tubes," boil up grated arrowroot tubers and eat by the tablespoonfuls, as if it were cereal.

Inflammation

MO: Break the hollow leaf stems of the the castor bean plant (*higuereta*), string them so that you have little necklaces of the appropriate size, and put them on the person's body. Good for any type of inflammation.

PV: Heat and chop up the leaf of the castor bean plant (*higuereta*) and make a poultice by mixing the chopped leaf with belladonna ointment. Then wrap it around the swollen, inflamed area. Good for any kind of inflammation, including for cows, when they are swollen after giving birth.

Insomnia

DB: Put a pastille of camphor (*alcanfor*) in a glass of water and place that glass under your bed before retiring.

ML: If a child can't sleep, give her a tea of sour orange leaves (*naranjo*).

Internal Pain

IV: Take a big handful of garlic weed (*anamú*), and mash it up in a mortar and pestle or put it in a blender with a cup and a half of water and strain. Take as needed.

Intestinal Gas

PA: Take a strong tea of anise (*anís*) seeds with coffee senna (*hedionda chiquita*) root and flowers.

OR Teas of basil (*albahaca*) alone or with anise seed or star anise (*anís estrellado*).

LF: Take a tea of coffee senna root (*hedionda chiquita*) boiled with slices of ginger (*jengibre dulce*).

CMS: Take teas of chamomile flowers (*manzanilla*).

Intestinal Parasites

B&CR: Cut some long slits into a just-harvested green papaya. Then, with a teaspoon, collect the white latex that seeps out of the cuts. Take a teaspoonful or two a day, always on an empty stomach. (Since the latex is caustic, dilute it a bit with juice.) Within three days you will have eliminated the parasites.

OR Place a clove of raw garlic in the rectum.

MO: Purslane (*verdolaga*) tea can be given to children to avoid their getting worms.

GS: Wormseed (*pazote*) tea is the best remedy, but it does stink. So hold your nose when you drink it, and the worms will leave your body in droves!

CVS: Drink the juice of the wormseed (*pazote*) plant on an empty stomach, a tablespoon at a time.

Kidney Pain & Inflammation

JS: Boil up a good deal of common plantain (*llantén*)—one part leaves to three parts water—for about twenty minutes, then strain it and use that water for a sitz bath. It cools, cleanses and alleviates inflammation.

PV&BV: Cut a "leaf" of the spineless (*tuna*) cactus into two flat slices. Then roast them and when they've cooled off, place them on the person's lower back over the kidneys and cover with a towel.

PA: For pain in the kidneys, make a poultice of the leaves of *baquiña cerrada*. First warm and "tenderize" each leaf with the steam of your teapot, then rub cooking oil or camphor ointment on top of them, and place over the kidneys. Cover with a towel and allow the oil or ointment to seep into the skin.

GS & MO: For kidney stones, take teas of *Juana la blanca* or *la baquiña cerrada*. Drink freely of *baquiña cerrada* but don't take *Juana la blanca* for more than three days in a row.

DC: For kidney stones, boil common plantain (*llantén*), *baquiña cerrada*, and *Juana la blanca* up together and strain. Serve every morning with the water of an entire coconut.

PS: Drink teas of mallow (*malva*), which are very cooling.
OR Drink lots of coconut water.

BV: Drink teas of amaranth (*blero*) and/or *cohitre blanco*.
OR Boil up a "leaf" of spineless (*tuna*) cactus, a little handful of *paletaria* and another little handful of black nightshade (*mata gallina*) in a litre of water for 20–25 minutes. Drink throughout the day.

Medicated Ointment/Oil for Poultices, Rubs, etc.

PA: Melt a five-ounce jar of Vaseline in a little saucepan over a low flame. Then mash two little blocks of camphor (*alcanfor*) until they're just powder, and add that powder to the Vaseline on the stove. When it's all dissolved, let it cool a little and then put it all back into the same Vaseline jar.

OR Add the camphor to cooking oil as it is heated upon the stove. If you want it to take a solid consistency, add grated paraffin or bees' wax to the oil as it cooks.

Menstrual Irregularities

JP: Boil up the root of coffee senna (*hedionda*) and take as tea. Brings on and normalizes menstruation.

JS: *Salvia* leaf tea corrects a "cold" womb condition.

PA: For menstrual pain, boil up the paper-like peel and ends of a couple of heads of garlic and drink as tea.

MO: Rue (*ruda*)* tea and broadleaf coriander (*culantro del monte* teas)* regulate the cycle and alleviate menstrual pain.

AND Garlic weed (*anamú*)* tea brings on the period.

PV: Take teas of rue (*ruda*)* and fennel (*hinojo*).

PS: Rue (*ruda*)* teas are very good for pains and problems of a woman's reproductive system.

CV: *Yerba Luisa** and *salvia* bring on a late period.

*Use these herbs with caution. May cause abortion.

Muscle Cramps

PV: For leg cramps and other body pains, roast some bitter ginger (*gengibre amargo*) until soft, then let cool. Mash two or three handfuls of ginger and add to 1 litre of alcoholated rubbing solution (*alcoholado*). As it sits, it gets stronger.

BV: Boil up the leaves of annato (*achiote*) and soak legs and feet in the warm liquid for muscle spasms.

OR Rub fresh (warm) urine into a cramped leg or foot.

BS: Rub corn silk into the cramped area.

Peace of Mind

DC: Pray for guidance and live gratefully, always carrying with you a symbol of thanks in your thoughts.

FB: Tend a home garden of vegetables, fruits and herbs. Enjoy the rewards of your labor and share with neighbors.

Pests

AC: To get rid of ticks, put all the *poleo* that fits—leaves without stems—into a bucket of water. The stronger the better, but don't boil it; simply leave the *poleo* there to steep from one day to the next; then you pour it in and around the doghouse or wherever the ticks are. The water has a strong smell, and the ticks will move on quickly.

CR: Cockroaches hate *poleo*! Put two or three branches of it in every corner throughout your home, and they'll just disappear.

BV: To get rid of fleas, lice, ticks and other pests, mix *Aguarrás* (a petroleum distillate used for rubdowns, available in pharmacies) with undiluted ammonia solution and mop the house with it.

ML: To keep moths, cockroaches and other pests away, put mashed-up pieces of *pacholí* root in drawers and closets.

Skin

irritation

PV: For itching problems, bathe in a solution of *cundeamor* or palma Christi (*higuereta*).

MO: To make a skin powder for heat rash, diaper rash and other irritations, grate arrowroot tubers (*maranta*) and dust with the silky starch.

B&CR: Crush the juice from the long, thick stems of comfrey (*consuelda mayor*) and use the juice as an ointment.

PV: For heat rash, drink *paletaria* tea. It's cooling, and especially effective for children's skin irritations.

to toughen

GS: For manual laborers: at night, work a tallow stick (*sebo Flandes*) into your hands. The next day, the skin on your hands will be hard and strong.

BV: To fit into tight shoes without getting corns and blisters, rub feet with tallow (*sebo Flandes*) the night before wearing the shoes, and then again immediately before and after wearing them.

for sunburn

PV: Cut a leaf of aloe vera (*sábila*) and pass the inside gel over the skin as if it were a lotion.

skin fungus

PA: Fill a bottle with fresh *cundeamor* and cover it all with three parts cooking oil and one part rubbing alcohol. Leave it for a few days so that the medicinal qualities and color of the plant can seep into the liquid. Apply it to the affected area as often as needed.

MO: Boil up some *cundeamor* and when the water is a deep green color, let it cool and apply it frequently.

BR&CR: Pick some stinging nettle leaves (*ortiga brava*) using gloves or a towel so as not to get stung, then use a mortar and pestle or a rolling pin to crush them. Place the crushed leaves and juice in water, and leave them there for three or four hours. Later, strain the water and keep it in the refrigerator. Every hour (at least six or seven times a day), wash the ailing area with the nettle water and let it dry in the air, without rubbing.

ringworm

CM: Cut a 6 or 8" piece of the trunk of dumb cane (*rábano cimarrón*) lengthwise and put some salt into the cut. (Three or four large salt grains will do, but you have to smash them up first.) Leave it all outside overnight so that it will absorb the cool, damp night air. During that time, the salt dissolves into the liquid from the cane, and in the morning you paint the ringworm with that liquid using a feather. It burns a little but that's how ringworm is cured.

BV: Mix squash resins in equal parts with the crushed leaves of the ringworm tree (*talantro*) and apply as a poultice.

IL: Mash up the leaves of the ringworm tree (*talantro*), and apply the juice all over the affected area, as often as needed.

Stomach Ulcers

IV: Every day, wash two handfuls of *cohitre blanco*, and place in a large mortar and pestle. Work it till the juice comes out, then boil both fiber and juice in a litre of water over a low flame for twenty minutes or so. Strain and take it three times a day: hot, warm, and cool, without sugar; a bit of honey may be used.

MOS: Boil a peeled, white onion for twenty minutes, and drink the water twice a day for ten days.

PS: Toss a couple of handfuls of common plantain (*llantén*) in the blender with a cup of water. Add some black nightshade (*mata gallina*), and drink daily on an empty stomach.

MO: Boil up common plantain (*llantén*) with black nightshade (*mata gallina*) and drink throughout the day.

DB: Boil up some black nightshade (*yerba mora*) in milk, either alone or in combination with leaves of common plantain (*llantén*). Drink on a regular basis.

ML: Take teas of *tuatúa* leaf buds with black nightshade leaves (*mata gallina*) before meals.

Swollen Glands & Mumps

CM: Rub glands with tallow (*sebo de Flandes*).

Teeth & Gums
(people & animals)

ML: For toothache, rinse the mouth with *amoniaco* (a dilute ammonia solution sold in pharmacies).

AND For gum problems, chop up a peeled leaf of aloe vera (*sábila*) and leave in water over night. Use as a mouthwash twice daily.

OR If you have false teeth, place a piece of sage leaf between gums and teeth and change daily. The juice then has a chance to massage the gums during the entire day.

AND When a child is teething, a little tea of *tuatúa* leaf buds will relieve him.

AC: If you don't have a toothbrush handy, place the leaf of the native lentil (*gandul*) against your gums and rub as if it were a little brush.

PV: Make a little packet of lemon grass (*limoncillo*) root and pass it over your gums as if it were a toothbrush. It freshens up the breath and makes your mouth feel great.

CM: For infection, rinse with hot salt water for long periods of time at every opportunity.

TR: For a tooth/gum infection, swish a "tea" of the boiled root of *moriviví* in your mouth as often as needed. And if the tooth is loose, this will help it come out.

PC: For toothache, rinse your mouth with a "tea" made from the leaves of the *guayacán*.

BV: After losing a tooth, place salt in the hollow where the tooth was. Will cleanse and cut the bleeding fast.

OR If there is hemorrhage, wash a bud of *salvia*, chew it up, and hold it in place on the gum itself. Will coagulate blood and alleviate pain.

CM: For loose teeth in cows, squeeze everything out of a lemon (some people roast their lemons first) and add some salt and sugar. Then rub it along the cow's gums, and don't give them water right away. If you don't have lemons around, you can use iodine. That tightens their teeth right up.

Throat Problems

AC: Gargle with lemon juice in warm salt water. The salt cleanses the throat, and the lemon has vitamin C.

CM: Drink *salvia* tea or chew the young leaf buds.

OR For serious throat problems, squeeze some lemon juice into a cup with a little water and add some white vinegar and salt. Heat it up and start gargling with it as hot as you can take it every once in a while, all through the day and night.

Udder Congestion (cows, goats, etc.)

GS: If your cow has milk balls in her udder, boil up some palma Christi plant (*higuereta*) in a big tub. Then, after it's boiled long enough so that the water has taken on the color of the leaves, skim off the foam. The next day, use those same leaves as towels and wash the udder completely with that liquid. Do it three times a day, with lots of strength, and you'll see plenty of milk as the balls disappear.

Urinary Tract Inflammation

CM: Make a tea of *prenetaria* mixed with spineless (*tuna*) cactus and drink throughout the day.

OR Make a simple tisane of *prenetaria*. Just wash the plant, add it to a jar of water and, after it's been sitting for some hours, drink throughout the day, as much as you want.

MO: Boil the leaves of mallow (*malva*) and black nightshade (*mata gallina*) in a litre of water; you can add some *paletaria* and spineless (*tuna*) cactus too. Take a cupful of this tea at least twice every day, and always at night. It usually cures completely, but you have to continue with the remedy for a while.

PV: Take strong teas of rue (*ruda*).

Uterine Inflammation

JP: After boiling a handful of castor bean plant (*ricino*) leaves in a large pot for 15 minutes, strain the liquid and pour it into warm bath water in a tub big enough to sit in. Sit there for ten or fifteen minutes or until you feel better.

JS: Boil up some wild eggplant (*berenjena cimarrona*) leaves. Then just sit for a while in that water, while it's fairly warm.

OR Boil up some mallow (*malva*) leaves, and after the water has cooled off a bit, add some Epsom salts. Sit in that water for as long as you can.

MO: Boil up the leaves of *campana* and use as a vaginal wash.

PS: Drink teas of mallow (*malva*) leaves.

Warming "Pleasure" Drinks

PV: Try a tea of marjoram (*mejorana*) with ginger (*jengibre dulce*), elder (*saúco*) and honey.

OR Mash up some ginger and boil it in a little bit of water for ten to fifteen minutes. Then mix that water with hot milk and add sugar to taste. Delicious!

Warts

ML: Wrap the mashed pulp of the tuberose (*azucena*) root on the warts with a cloth.

B&CR: Pick a few leaves of the poinsettia plant (*pascua*) and apply the milky juice that flows from the cut areas to the warts. They'll disappear after just four or five applications.

Medicinal Plants

by Name and Family

INDEX I

INDEX II, on p. 231 is organized in alphabetical order, by English.

PUERTO RICAN / SPANISH NAME(S)	LATIN NAME(S)	ENGLISH NAME(S)	BOTANICAL FAMILY
achicoria, chicoria	Cichorium intybus	chicory	Compositae
achiote, bija	Bixa orellana	annato	Bixaceae
afilerillo, cabellos de ángel, tente en el aire	Cassytha filiformis	love vine	Lauraceae
aguacate	Persea americana	avocado	Lauraceae
ajo	Allium sativum	garlic	Liliaceae
ajonjolí	Sesamum indicum	sesame	Pedaliaceae
albahaca (blanca)	Ocimum basilicum	basil	Labiatae

PUERTO RICAN / SPANISH NAME(S)	LATIN NAME(S)	ENGLISH NAME(S)	BOTANICAL FAMILY
alcanfor	Cinnamomum camphora	camphor	Lauraceae
eucalipto	Eucalyptus globulus	eucalyptus	Myrtaceae
almendra	Terminalia catappa	tropical almond	Combretaceae
altamisa, artemisa	Ambrosia peru-viana	mugwort	Compositae
anacagüita	Sterculia apetala	Panama tree	Sterculiaceae
anamú	Petiveria alliacea	garlic weed, congo root	Phytolaccaceae
anís, anís en grano	Pimpinella anisum	anise seed	Umbelliferae
anís de estrella	Illicium anisatum	star anise	Magnoliaceae
árnica	Arnica montana	arnica	Compositae
azucena (del Caribe)	Polianthes tuberosa	tuberose	Amaryllidaceae
bálsamo, péndula	Citharexylum fruticosum		Rubiaceae
baquiña cerrada	Lepianthes peltatum	monkey's hand	Piperaceae
berenjena cimarrona	Solanum torvum	wild eggplant	Solanaceae
berro, berro de agua	Nasturtium officinale	watercress	Papaveraceae
blero	Amaranthus viridis	amaranth	Amaranthaceae

PUERTO RICAN / SPANISH NAME(S)	LATIN NAME(S)	ENGLISH NAME(S)	BOTANICAL FAMILY
botón de cadete, molinillo	Leonotis nepetifolia	lion's ear	Labiatae
bruja, siempreviva	Kalanchoë pinnatum	life plant	Crassulaceae
cabellos de ángel, tente en el aire, afilerillo	Cassytha filiformis	love vine	Lauraceae
cadillo, caíllo, pata de perro	Urena lobata (sinuata)	bur	Malvaceae
café	Coffea arabica	coffee	Rubiaceae
caimito	Chrysophyllum cainito	star apple	Sapotaceae
campana, campano	Datura suaveolens	moon plant	Solanaceae
cañafístula	Cassia fistula	purging cassia	Caesalpiniaceae
canario (amarillo)	Allamanda cathartica	yellow allamanda	Apocynaceae
canela	Cinnamomum zeylanicum	cinammon	Lauraceae
canela (del país) canelillo	Licaria salicifolia	Puerto Rican cinammon	Lauraceae
cariaquillo (legítimo)	Lantana camara	red, yellow sage	Verbenaceae
cebolla	Allium cepa	onion	Liliaceae
ceiba	Ceiba pentandra	silk-cotton tree	Bombacaceae
cilantro, cilantrillo	Coriandrum sativum	coriander	Umbelliferae

PUERTO RICAN / SPANISH NAME(S)	LATIN NAME(S)	ENGLISH NAME(S)	BOTANICAL FAMILY
clavo de especia clavo dulce	Syzygium aromaticum	clove	Myrtaceae
cohitre blanco	Campelia zanonia	white French weed	Commelinaceae
col blanco	Brassica oleracea	cabbage	Cruciferae
consuelda mayor	Symphytum officinalis	comfrey	Boraginaceae
corazón	Annona reticulata	custard apple, Bullock's heart	Annonaceae
culantro del monte, recao	Eryngium foetidum	Puerto Rican coriander, broadleaf coriander	Umbelliferae
cundeamor	Momordica charantia	wild balsam apple	Cucurbitaceae
curía, tilo	Justicia pectoralis		Acanthaceae
chicoria, achicoria	Cichorium intybus	chicory	Compositae
chucho, cocuisa lengua de vaca, sansiviera	Sansevieria metallica	snake plant, African bowstring, Guana tail, bowstring hemp	Liliaceae
escobilla	Vernonia sericea (?)		Compositae
eucalipto eucalipto (medicinal)	Eucalyptus globulus, Eucalyptus resinifera	eucalyptus, Kino gum eucalyptus	Myrtaceae

PUERTO RICAN / SPANISH NAME(S)	LATIN NAME(S)	ENGLISH NAME(S)	BOTANICAL FAMILY
gandul	Cajanus cajan	native lentil pigeon pea	Leguminosae
geranio (oloroso)	Geranium odoratissium	fragrant geranium	Geraniaceae
gran señora		bitter mint	Labiatae
guaco	Mikania cordifolia	guaco	Compositae
guanábana	Annona muricata	soursop	Annonaceae
guayabo	Psidium guajava	guava	Myrtaceae
guayacán, guayaco	Guaiacum officinale		Zygophyllaceae
hedionda (chiquita)	Senna occidentalis	coffee senna	Caesalpiniaceae
hicaco	Chrysobalanus icaco	coco plum	Chripobalanceae
higüera	Crescentia cujete	calabash, gourd	Bignoniaceae
higuereta, ricino	Ricinus communis	castor bean plant, palma Christi	Euphorbiaceae
higuillo oloroso	Piper marginatum		Piperaceae
hinojo	Foeniculum vulgare	fennel	Umbelliferae
ipecacuana díctamo real	Pedilanthus tithymaloides	slipper plant	Euphorbiaceae
jagua, genipa	Genipa americana	genipap	Rubiaceae

PUERTO RICAN / SPANISH NAME(S)	LATIN NAME(S)	ENGLISH NAME(S)	BOTANICAL FAMILY
jengibre amargo	Zingiber zerumbet	bitter ginger	Zingiberaceae
jengibre dulce, jengibre del país	Zingiber officinale	ginger	Zingiberaceae
jobo	Spondias dulcis	yellow mombin	Anacardiaceae
Juana la blanca	Borreria laevis	iron grass	Rubiaceae
lechosa, papaya	Carica papaya	papaya	Caricaceae
limón	Citrus limon	lemon	Rutaceae
limoncillo	Cymbopogon citratus	lemon grass	Gramineae
llantén	Plantago major, Plantago lanceolata, Plantago m & p	broad-leaf plantain, narrow-leaf plantain, common plantain	Plantaginaceae
madera del país			
maga	Montezuma grandiflora	maga wood	Malvaceae
malá (blanca)	Senecio aizoides	malá	Compositae
malagueta	Pimenta racemosa	bay rum	Myrtaceae
malva	Malachra capitata	mallow	Malvaceae
mango, mangó	Mangifera indica	mango	Anacardiaceae

PUERTO RICAN / SPANISH NAME(S)	LATIN NAME(S)	ENGLISH NAME(S)	BOTANICAL FAMILY
manzanilla	Anthemis nobilis, Wedelia trilobata Euphoria didyma	chamomile	Compositae Compositae Sapindaceae
maranta, yuquilla, amaranta, pitisilén	Maranta arundinacea	arrowroot	Marantaceae
mata dulce yerba dulce	Lippia dulcis	sweet verbena	Verbenaceae
mata gallina yerba mora	Solanum americanum	black nightshade	Solanaceae
maya	Bromelia pingüin		Bromeliaceae
mejorana	Origanum marjorana	marjoram	Labiatae
menta	Mentha piperata, Mentha spicata	peppermint, spearmint	Labiatae
morera	Morus nigra	(black) mulberry	Moraceae
moriviví, mimosa	Mimosa pudica	sensitive plant	Mimosaceae
naranja(o)	Citrus aurantium	sour orange	Rutaceae
ñame	Dioscorea alata	yam	Dioscoreaceae
nemoscá, nuez moscada nemocá	Myristica fragrans	nutmeg	Myristicaceae

PUERTO RICAN / SPANISH NAME(S)	LATIN NAME(S)	ENGLISH NAME(S)	BOTANICAL FAMILY
nemoscá, nemocá, nuez moscada del país	Ocotea moschata	Puerto Rican nutmeg	Myristicaceae
orégano (chiquito) orégano del país	Lippia micromera	Puerto Rican oregano	Verbenaceae
ortiga (brava)	Urera baccifera	giant stinging nettle	Urticaceae
pacholí, pachulí baúl de pobre	Vetiveria zizanioides	vetiver, Caribbean pachouli	Gramineae
pajuil, cajuil marañon	Anacardium occidentale	cashew	Anacardiaceae
paletaria, prenetaria, parietaria, alumbre, frescura	Peperomia pellucida		Piperaceae
palma de coco cocotero, coco	Cocos nucifera	coconut palm	Palmaceae
palma real palma de yaguas	Roystonea borinquena	Puerto Rican royal palm	Palmaceae
papa	Solanum tuberosum	potato	Solanaceae
papaya, lechosa	Carica papaya	papaya	Caricaceae
parcha, pasionaria	Passiflora edulis	passion fruit	Passifloraceae
pascua	Euphorbia pulcherrima	poinsettia	Euphorbiaceae

PUERTO RICAN / SPANISH NAME(S)	LATIN NAME(S)	ENGLISH NAME(S)	BOTANICAL FAMILY
pata de perro cadillo, caíllo	Urena lobata (sinuata)	bur	Malvaceae
pazote	Chenopodium ambrosioides	wormseed	Chenopodiaceae
pimienta Angola boca de dragón	Alpinia zerumbet	shell plant, shell flower	Zingiberaceae
poleo	Lippia stoechadifolia		Verbenaceae
prenetaria, paletaria parietaria, alumbre frescura	Peperomia pellucida		Piperaceae
pringamosa	Tragia volubilis	stinging vine	Euphorbiaceae
quinino de pobre	Phyllanthus niruri	gale of the wind	Euphorbiaceae
rábano cimarrón	Dieffenbachia seguine	dumb cane	Araceae
recao, culantro del monte	Eryngium foetidum	Puerto Rican coriander, broadleaf coriander	Umbelliferae
ricino, higuereta	Ricinus communis	castor bean plant, palma Christi	Euphorbiaceae
roble amarillo	Tabebuia rufescens		Bignoniaceae
romero	Rosmarinus officinalis	rosemary	Labiatae
rompecota			

PUERTO RICAN / SPANISH NAME(S)	LATIN NAME(S)	ENGLISH NAME(S)	BOTANICAL FAMILY
rosa (cienhojas)	Rosa centifolia	fairy rose	Rosaceae
ruda	Ruta chalepensis	rue, garden rue	Rutaceae
sábila, sávila závila	Aloe vera	aloe (vera)	Liliaceae
sacabuche	Physalis angulata, Physalis eggersii, Physalis peruviana, Physalis pubescens,	ground cherry	Solanaceae
	Physalis turbinata	husk tomato	
salvia (olorosa)	Pluchea symphytifolia	sweet scent	Compositae
sanguinaria, sangría	Rhoeo spathacea	oyster plant	Commelinaceae
santa María	Eupatorium odoratum,	bitter bush	Compositae
	Lantana involucrata		Verbenaceae
saúco (blanco)	Sambucus mexicana	elder	Caprifoliaceae
saúco amarillo	Tecoma stans	yellow elder	Bignoniaceae
sueldaconsuelda	Anredera leptostachys	Madeira vine	Basellaceae
tabaco	Nicotiana tabacum	tobacco	Solanaceae
talantro, talantalán, talantrillo	Senna alata	ringworm tree	Caesalpiniaceae

PUERTO RICAN / SPANISH NAME(S)	LATIN NAME(S)	ENGLISH NAME(S)	BOTANICAL FAMILY
tamarindo	Tamarindus indica	tamarind	Caesalpiniaceae
tártago, piñón	Jatropha curcas	physic nut	Euphorbiaceae
tautúa, tuatúa, higuereta cimarrona	Jatropha gossypifolia		Euphorbiaceae
tente en el aire, cabellos de angel, afilerillo	Cassytha filiformis	love vine	Lauraceae
tilo (árbol)	Tilia europea (platyphillos)	linden	Tiliaceae
tilo (mata), curía	Justicia pectoralis		Acanthaceae
tomate	Lycopersicon lycopersicum	tomato	Solanaceae
toronjil	Melissa officinalis	lemon balm	Labiatae
tuatúa, tautúa, higuereta cimarrona	Jatropha gossypifolia		Euphorbiaceae
tuna	Opuntia ficus-indica	Spineless tuna cactus, Indian fig cactus	Cactaceae
valeriana	Valeriana scandens	valerian	Valerianaceae
vara prieta			
verbena	Stachytarpheta jamaicensis	Caribbean vervain	Verbenaceae
verdolaga	Portulaca oleracea	purslane	Portulacaceae

PUERTO RICAN / SPANISH NAME(S)	LATIN NAME(S)	ENGLISH NAME(S)	BOTANICAL FAMILY
yapaná jazmín hediondo, flor de muerto	Clerodendron philippinum	wild jessamine	Verbenaceae
yerba cangá	Ludwigia octovalvis		Onagraceae
yerba dulce mata dulce	Lippia dulcis	sweet verbena	Verbenaceae
yerba (de) guinea, gramalote, yerba Borinquen	Panicum maximum	guinea grass	Gramineae
yerba Luisa	Aloysia triphylla	lemon vervain	Verbenaceae
yerba mora, mata gallina	Solanum americanum	black nightshade	Solanaceae

Please note:

Despite the author's efforts, some plants have not been identified completely. In most cases, English names are lacking. In the cases of *gran señora, madera del país, rompecota,* and *vara prieta*, the plants named (and as observed or described by contributors) are not listed in any botanical reference known to the author. In the case of *escobilla*, the plant's soapy quality, described by natives of Mayagüez, is not attributed to the plants catalogued as *escobilla* in botanical literature.

Knowledgable readers are encouraged to write the author with information leading to the complete identification of such plants. Accordingly, future editions of this work will include an updated index.

Medicinal Plants

by Name and Family

INDEX II

ENGLISH NAME(S)	PUERTO RICAN / SPANISH NAME(S)	LATIN NAME(S)	BOTANICAL FAMILY
aloe (vera)	sábila, sávila závila	Aloe vera	Liliaceae
amaranth	blero	Amaranthus viridis	Amaranthaceae
anise (seed)	anís, anís en grano	Pimpinella anisum	Umbelliferae
annato	achiote, bija	Bixa orellana	Bixaceae
arnica	árnica	Arnica montana	Compositae
arrowroot	maranta, yuquilla, amaranta, pitsilén	Maranta arundinacea	Marantaceae
avocado	aguacate	Persea americana	Lauraceae
basil	albahaca (blanca)	Ocimum basilicum	Labiatae
bay rum	malagueta	Pimenta racemosa	Myrtaceae

ENGLISH NAME(S)	PUERTO RICAN / SPANISH NAME(S)	LATIN NAME(S)	BOTANICAL FAMILY
bitter bush	santa María	Eupatorium odoratum Lantana involucrata	Compositae Verbenaceae
bitter ginger	jengibre amargo	Zingiber zerumbet	Zingiberaceae
bitter mint	gran señora		Labiatae
black night-shade	yerba mora, mata gallina	Solanum americanum	Solanaceae
broad-leaf coriander, Puerto Rican coriander	recáo, culantro del monte	Eryngium foetidum	Umbelliferae
bur	cadillo, caíllo, pata de perro	Urena lobata (sinuata)	Malvaceae
cabbage	col blanco	Brassica oleracea	Cruciferae
calabash, gourd	higüera	Crescentia cujete	Bignoniaceae
camphor eucalyptus	alcanfor	Cinnamomum camphora Eucalyptus globulus	Lauraceae Myrtaceae
Caribbean pachouli, vetiver	pacholí, pachulí, baúl de pobre	Vetiveria zizanioides	Gramineae
(Caribbean) vervain	verbena	Stachytarpheta jamaicensis	Verbenaceae
cashew	pajuil, cajuil, marañon	Anacardium occidentale	Anacardiaceae

ENGLISH NAME(S)	PUERTO RICAN / SPANISH NAME(S)	LATIN NAME(S)	BOTANICAL FAMILY
castor bean plant, palma Christi	higuereta, ricino	Ricinus communis	Euphorbiaceae
chamomile	manzanilla	Anthemis nobilis Wedelia trilobata Euphoria didyma	Compositae Compositae Sapindaceae
chicory	chicoria, achicoria	Cichorium intybus	Compositae
cinammon	canela	Cinnamomum zeylanicum	Lauraceae
clove	clavo de especia, clavo dulce	Syzygium aromaticum	Myrtaceae
coco plum	hicaco	Chrysobalanus icaco	Chripobalanceae
coconut palm	palma de coco, cocotero, coco	Cocos nucifera	Palmaceae
coffee	café	Coffea arabica	Rubiaceae
coffee senna	hedionda (chiquita)	Senna occidentalis	Caesalpiniaceae
comfrey	consuelda mayor	Symphytum officinalis	Boraginaceae
common plantain, broadleaf plantain narrow-leaf plantain	llantén	Plantago m & l Plantago mayor Plantago lanceolata	Plantaginaceae

ENGLISH NAME(S)	PUERTO RICAN / SPANISH NAME(S)	LATIN NAME(S)	BOTANICAL FAMILY
coriander	cilantro, cilantrillo	Coriandrum sativum	Umbelliferae
custard apple, Bullock's heart	corazon	Annona reticulata	Annonaceae
dumb cane	rábano cimarrón	Dieffenbachia seguine	Araceae
elder	saúco (blanco)	Sambucus mexicana	Caprifoliaceae
eucalyptus	eucalipto, alcanfor, eucalipto medicinal	Eucalyptus globulus	Myrtaceae
fairy rose	rosa (cienhojas)	Rosa centifolia	Rosaceae
fennel	hinojo	Foeniculum vulgare	Umbelliferae
fragrant geranium	geranio (oloroso)	Geranium odoratissium	Geraniaceae
gale of the wind	quinino de pobre	Phyllanthus niruri	Euphorbiaceae
garlic	ajo	Allium sativum	Liliaceae
garlic weed congo root	anamú	Petiveria alliacea	Phytolaccaceae
genipap	jagua, genipa	Genipa americana	Rubiaceae
giant stinging nettle	ortiga (brava)	Urera baccifera	Urticaceae
ginger, sweet ginger	jengibre dulce, jengibre del país	Zingiber officinale	Zingiberaceae
gourd, calabash	higüera	Crescentia cujete	Bignoniaceae

ENGLISH NAME(S)	PUERTO RICAN / SPANISH NAME(S)	LATIN NAME(S)	BOTANICAL FAMILY
ground cherry	sacabuche	Physalis angulata Physalis eggersii Physalis peruviana Physalis pubescens Physalis turbinata	Solanaceae
guaco	guaco	Mikania cordifolia	Compositae
guava	guayabo	Psidium guajava	Myrtaceae
guinea grass	yerba (de) guinea, gramalote, yerba Borinquen	Panicum maximum	Gramineae
iron grass	Juana la blanca	Borreria laevis	Rubiaceae
lemon	limón	Citrus limon	Rutaceae
lemon balm	toronjil	Melissa officinalis	Labiatae
lemon grass	limoncillo	Cymbolpogon citratus	Gramineae
lemon vervain	yerba Luisa	Aloysia triphylla	Verbenaceae
life plant	bruja, siempreviva	Kalanchoë pinnatum	Crassulaceae
linden	tilo (árbol)	Tilia europa (platyphillos)	Tiliaceae

ENGLISH NAME(S)	PUERTO RICAN / SPANISH NAME(S)	LATIN NAME(S)	BOTANICAL FAMILY
lion's ear	botón de cadete, molinillo	Leonotis nepetifolia	Labiatae
love vine	tente en el aire, cabellos de angel, afilerillo	Cassytha filiformis	Lauraceae
Madeira vine	sueldaconsuelda	Anredera leptostachys	Basellaceae
maga wood	maga	Montezuma grandiflora	Malvaceae
malá	malá (blanca)	Senecio aizoides	Compositae
mallow	malva	Malachra capitata	Malvaceae
mango	mango, mangó	Mangifera indica	Anacardiaceae
marjoram	mejorana	Origanum marjorana	Labiatae
monkey's hand	baquiña cerrada	Lepianthes peltatum	Piperaceae
moon plant	campana, campano	Datura suaveolens	Solanaceae
mugwort	altamisa, artemisa	Ambrosia peruviana	Compositae
mulberry (black)	morera	Morus nigra	Moraceae
native lentil pigeon pea	gandul	Cajanus cajun	Leguminosae
nutmeg	nemoscá, nemocá, nuez moscoda	Myristica fragrans	Myristicaceae

ENGLISH NAME(S)	PUERTO RICAN / SPANISH NAME(S)	LATIN NAME(S)	BOTANICAL FAMILY
onion	cebolla	Allium cepa	Liliaceae
oyster plant	sanguinaria, sangría	Rhoeo spathacea	Commelinaceae
palma Christi, castor bean plant	higuereta, ricino	Ricinus communis	Euphorbiaceae
Panama tree	anacagüita	Sterculia apetala	Sterculiaceae
papaya	papaya, lechosa	Carica papaya	Caricaceae
passion fruit	parcha, pasionaria	Passiflora edulis	Passifloraceae
peppermint	menta	Mentha piperata	Labiatae
pigeon pea, native lentil	gandul	Cajanus cajan	Leguminosae
poinsettia	pascua	Euphorbia pulcherrima	Euphorbiaceae
physic nut	tártago, piñón	Jatropha curcas	Euphorbiaceae
potato	papa	Solanum tuberosum	Solanaceae
Puerto Rican cinammon	canela (del país), canelillo	Licaria salicifolia	Lauraceae
Puerto Rican coriander, broadleaf coriander	culantro del monte, recao	Eryngium foetidum	Umbelliferae
Puerto Rican nutmeg	nemoscá, nemocá, nuez moscada del país	Ocotea moschata	Myristicaceae
Puerto Rican oregano	orégano (chiquito)	Lippia micromera	Verbenaceae

ENGLISH NAME(S)	PUERTO RICAN / SPANISH NAME(S)	LATIN NAME(S)	BOTANICAL FAMILY
Puerto Rican royal palm	palma real, palma de yaguas	Roystonea borinquena	Palmaceae
purging cassia	cañafístula	Cassia fistula	Caesalpiniaceae
purslane	verdolaga	Portulaca oleracea	Portulacaceae
red mint	yerba buena	Mentha nemorosa	Labiatae
red, yellow sage	cariaquillo (legítimo)	Lantana camara	Verbenaceae
ringworm tree	talantro, talantalán, talantrillo	Senna alata	Caesalpiniaceae
tohrosemary	romero	Rosmarinus officinalis	Labiatae
rue	ruda	Ruta chalepensis	Rutaceae
sensitive plant	moriviví, mimosa	Mimosa pudica	Mimosaceae
sesame	ajonjolí	Sesamum indicum	Pedaliaceae
shell flower, shell plant	pimienta Angola, boca de dragón	Alpinia zerumbet	Zingiberaceae
silk cotton tree	ceiba	Ceiba pentandra	Bombacaceae
slipper plant, ipecacuana, díctamo real	Pedilanthus tithymadloides	Euphorbiaceae	

ENGLISH NAME(S)	PUERTO RICAN / SPANISH NAME(S)	LATIN NAME(S)	BOTANICAL FAMILY
snake plant, African bowstring, Guana tail	chucho, cocuisa, lengua de vaca, sansiviera	Sansevieria metallica	Liliaceae
sour orange	naranja(o)	Citrus aurantium	Rutaceae
soursop	guanábana	Annona muricata	Annonaceae
spearmint	menta	Mentha spicata	Labiatae
spineless tuna cactus, Indian fig cactus	tuna	Opuntia ficus-indica	Cactaceae
star anise	anís de estrella	Illicium anisatum	Magnoliaceae
star apple	caimito	Chrysophyllum cainito	Sapotaceae
stinging vine	pringamosa	Tragia volubilis	Euphorbiaceae
sweet ginger ginger	jengibre dulce	Zingiber officinale	Zingiberaceae
sweet scent	salvia (olorosa)	Pluchea symphytifolia	Compositae
sweet verbena	mata dulce yerba dulce	Lippia dulcis	Verbenaceae
tamarind	tamarindo	Tamarindus indica	Caesalpiniaceae
tobacco	tabaco	Nicotiana tabacum	Solanaceae
tomato	tomate	Lycopersicon lycopersicum	Solanaceae

ENGLISH NAME(S)	PUERTO RICAN / SPANISH NAME(S)	LATIN NAME(S)	BOTANICAL FAMILY
tropical almond	almendra	Terminalia catappa	Combretaceae
tuberose	azucena (del Caribe)	Polianthes tuberosa	Amaryllidaceae
valerian	valeriana	Valeriana scandens	Valerianaceae
vetiver, Caribbean pachouli	pacholí, pachulí, baúl de pobre	Vitiveria zizanioides	Gramineae
watercress	berro de agua	Nasturtium officinale	Papaveraceae
white French weed	cohitre blanco	Campelia zanonia	Commelinaceae
wild balsam apple	cundeamor	Momordica charantia	Cucurbitaceae
wild eggplant	berenjena cimarrona	Solanum torvum	Solanaceae
wild jessamine	yapaná, jazmín, hediondo, flor de muerto	Clerodendron philippinum	Verbenaceae
wild zinnia	escopetón	Zinnia peruviana	Compositae
wormseed	pazote	Chenopodium ambrosioides	Chenopodiaceae
yam	ñame	Dioscorea alata	Dioscoreacea
yellow allamanda	canario (amarillo)	Allamanda cathartica	Apocynaceae
yellow mombin	jobo	Spondias dulcis	Anacardiaceae
yellow elder	saúco amarillo	Tacoma stans	Bignoniaceae
yellow, red sage	cariaquillo (legítimo)	Lantana camara	Verbenaceae

Spanish and Puerto Rican Words & Terms

A Glossary

Abuelita: an affectionate way of saying *abuela*, grandma.

Aceituna: olive.

Alcoholado: an analgesic and cooling infusion of herbs in dilute rubbing alcohol used for rubdowns and massages.

Apio: celeriac root.

Arroz con dulce: also known on the island as *arroz con coco*, this is a sliceable coconut rice pudding, sweet and seasoned with cloves, cinammon, ginger, vanilla, raisins and other delectables.

Arroz con gandules: a simple and most typical rice plate, prepared with local lentils, tomatoes, and local spices.

Arroz con pollo: chicken and rice, Puerto Rican style.

Bacalao con pana: salted codfish served with velvety-smooth, potato-like breadfruit.

Barrio: translated as "neighborhood" in urban North America. In Puerto Rico this word denotes a rural community.

Bendición: literally, "blessing." It usually takes the form of a hello and goodbye greeting such as "May God bless you and take care of you for me." Children traditionally ask for the *bendición* from their parents and other elders at every meeting and leavetaking.

Bomba, plena and *salsa*: *Bomba* and *plena* are African-derived musical forms developed in the coastal towns of Puerto Rico. Both are characterized by call and response song patterns and popular themes ranging from historical events and social commentary to discussion of the musical event in progress. *Bomba* is played with three barrel-shaped drums, one of which responds to song lyrics and the movements of a male dancer. *Plena* is played with four hand drums or *panderetas* and a *güiro*. *Salsa* or *mambo* is a popular dance form based on a complex of Afro-cuban rhythms, played by a full band of instruments including percussion, brass, piano, reeds, etc.

Campesina(o): often translated as "peasant," this word most accurately describes a rural person involved with working on the land; most often a farmer of some type.

Como Dios manda: as God intended.

Coquí: a small island frog which, during the night, sings a gentle, high-pitched version of its name. Native only to Puerto Rico—and reportedly unable to survive in any other environment—the *coquí* (*Eleutherodactylus coqui*) has become a symbol of the importance of maintaining the island's ecological balance and cultural integrity.

Dulce de coco: a candy-like sweet made from grated coconut, sugar and spices.

Espiritista: a diviner and spiritual healer, sometimes a medium. Very often, a member of a popular religious sect which holds meetings at special centers in order to do divination, healings and exorcisms involving communication with the world beyond.

Guaraguao: the broad-winged buzzard (*Buteo platypterus*), a large bird of prey.

Guarapo or *té, tesito* or *tesesito*: the traditional Puerto Rican *guarapo* or medicinal tea (actually, a decoction) is made more or less the following way (varying slightly from home to home). To a litre of boiling water, add one handful of well-rinsed, fresh plant material. Lower the heat, cover, and simmer for about fifteen minutes, or until the water takes on a deep color, usually green. According to several contributors, *guarapos* are usually drunk warm at night, and cool during the day. Refrigerated, they may be enjoyed instead of water, sugary sodas or other commercial beverages. It is usually